Healthy Villages
A guide for communities and community health workers

Guy Howard
Water, Engineering and Development Centre
Loughborough University, Loughborough, England

with

Claus Bogh
Bilharziasis Laboratory, Charlottenlund, Denmark

Greg Goldstein
Protection of the Human Environment
World Health Organization, Geneva, Switzerland

Joy Morgan
United Nations Children's Fund
Dhaka, Bangladesh

Annette Prüss
Protection of the Human Environment
World Health Organization, Geneva, Switzerland

Rod Shaw
Water, Engineering and Development Centre
Loughborough University, Loughborough, England

Joanna Teuton
Centre for Applied Psychology
University of Leicester, Leicester, England

World Health Organization
Geneva
2002

WHO Library Cataloguing-in-Publication Data

Howard, Guy
   Healthy villages : a guide for communities and community health workers / Guy Howard with Claus
   Bogh . . . [et al.]

   1.Rural health services – handbooks   2.Community health services – handbooks   3.Community health
   aides – handbooks   I.Bogh, Claus   II.Title

   ISBN 92 4 154553 4   (NLM Classification: WA 390)

The designations employed and the presentation of the material in this publication do not imply the expression of any opinion whatsoever on the part of the Secretariat of the World Health Organization concerning the legal status of any country, territory, city or area or of its authorities, or concerning the delimitation of its frontiers or boundaries.

The mention of specific companies or of certain manufacturers' products does not imply that they are recommended by the World Health Organization in preference to others of a similar nature that are not mentioned. Errors and omissions excepted, the names of proprietary products are distinguished by initial capital letters.

The authors alone are responsible for the views expressed in this publication.

Designed by WHO Graphics
TYPESET IN HONG KONG
PRINTED IN MALTA

2001/13840—Best-set/Interprint—7500

Contents

Foreword

Document aims and target audience

This guide was developed to support the Healthy Villages approach for improving the health of rural communities. It provides local community leaders with a model of the type of information they may need to consider in their roles as current or prospective managers of a Healthy Villages project. Community leaders include not only elected officials, but also the health staff, respected elders and others who work to improve the health of rural communities. We outline the type of information that Healthy Villages managers could provide to their communities, as well as the basis for developing material that is specific to regions or to entire countries. Because this guide was designed to be used in many different countries, it is likely that modifications will be required at local levels to ensure that local conditions and practices are taken into account.

It is recognized that many excellent locally-developed solutions for village health problems are already being practised. This guide is not intended as a global prescription for promoting improved health in rural communities, but rather as source material from which readers can develop local solutions to local problems. The purpose of this guide, therefore, is to provide a model of the type of information and approaches for promoting healthier villages that readers can use when implementing village-level activities.

The Healthy Villages project

Many countries are developing stronger partnerships between the health sector and local government organizations to promote local "settings" initiatives for health. A Healthy Villages project assists in this by putting concepts such as hygiene education, environmental health, health promotion and environmental protection into action in rural communities. A Healthy Villages project enables a village to mobilize the human and financial resources needed to address many health and quality-of-life issues. The process works as a communication strategy that develops political and popular health awareness and support for health issues.

Settings are major social structures that provide ways of reaching defined populations. Each setting in a village has a unique set of members, authorities, rules and participating organizations, each with interests in different aspects of the village life. For example, work settings include agriculture and small-scale industry; other settings include the food-market, the housing setting or the school setting. Generally, these structures are organized for purposes other than health. Interactions are frequent and sustained in these settings and are characterized by patterns of formal and informal membership and communication. These qualities create efficiencies in time and resources for health education programming, and offer more access and greater potential for social influence.

Villages are often defined in terms of arbitrary administrative definitions. A village may be a small group of people living in a settlement who practise subsistence agriculture, with no specialization or division of labour, and who are isolated from national development agencies. A village may also be a large and differentiated conurbation where some people work in agriculture, some work in small-scale industries and others provide education, health care, administration and a variety of services. This guide is directed towards the larger and more differentiated village. It is also recognized that many villages do not operate independently from cities, in that cities require sustained interaction with rural communities for their food and natural resources (including land for waste disposal). Often, too, the district agencies that set policy and administer the villages are located in cities. Under these circumstances, a Healthy Villages programme has a greater chance of success if the linked city is participating in a similar type of programme for cities—a Healthy Cities Programme[1]—and if the district-level staff implement Healthy Villages as part of the health policy for all the towns and villages in the district.

---

[1] Werna E et al. *Healthy city projects in developing countries: an international approach to local problems.* London, Earthscan, 1998.

Acknowledgements

The preparation of this guide was coordinated by the Water, Sanitation and Health programme, Protection of the Human Environment Department, of the World Health Organization in support of the Healthy Villages Programme. Its preparation was initiated and led by Annette Prüss.

The authors gratefully acknowledge the contributions of the participants in the following two expert consultations organized by WHO's Regional Office for the Eastern Mediterranean:

- Regional Consultation on the development of technical guidelines and integrated environmental management norms for Healthy Villages, Tabriz, Islamic Republic of Iran, June 1998
- Inter-regional Consultation on Healthy Villages, Damascus, Syria, October 1999.

The authors would also like to thank the staff from WHO Headquarters and WHO Regional Office for the Eastern Mediterranean for their comments on the content and style of the guide. In particular thanks go to Kumars Khosh-Chashm for his support.

Finally, the authors would like to acknowledge the editorial work of Kevin Farrell.

CHAPTER 1

Introduction

Many factors determine the health both of individuals and of the communities in which they live. These factors include income, social relationships, access to and use of basic services such as water supply and sanitation, the quality of available health services, individual responsibility and the quality of the environment. Consequently, public health interventions designed to reduce the risk of ill-health and promote feelings of well-being in a community must consider many social and environmental factors. These factors will vary in importance between communities, because of differences in the current services, facilities, priorities and needs of the communities, and because communities change over time. If health interventions are needed in several areas, they may need to be prioritized before they are implemented. Several programmes, such as primary health care or the Basic Development Needs programme,[1] address the factors that influence the health and well-being of communities. Advice on these programmes is available from a number of sources (see Annexes 1 and 2).

This guide focuses on the different health interventions that support the development of healthy communities. Many of the interventions require outside support to the communities, such as from local and national governments and nongovernmental organizations (NGOs). However, the communities themselves also play an important role in identifying problems, defining solutions and setting priorities. Often, communities will also need to participate directly in implementing solutions and in sustaining the improvements made. Indeed, many interventions require commitments from individual community members and households, in addition to commitments from the broader community. Frequently, the most important element in promoting health is to ensure that everyone has access to services.

---

[1] Abdullatif AA. Basic development needs approach in the Eastern Mediterranean Region. *Mediterranean Health Journal*, 1999, 5:168–176.

Characteristics of a healthy community

- The physical environment is clean and safe.
- The environment meets everyone's basic needs.
- The environment promotes social harmony and actively involves everyone.
- There is an understanding of the local health and environment issues.
- The community participates in identifying local solutions to local problems.
- Community members have access to varied experiences, interaction and communication.
- The health services are accessible and appropriate.
- The historical and cultural heritage is promoted and celebrated.
- There is a diverse and innovative economy.
- There is a sustainable use of available resources for all.

The purposes of this guide are:

- To help community leaders and people who work with rural communities identify problems that affect health.
- To outline possible solutions to these problems.
- To help in the setting of priorities that will lead to a healthier community.

During the development of the draft version of this guide many workshops and discussions were held with public health practitioners. Based on these discussions, it is expected that health department officials will find the guide a valuable tool for their community health work, and may translate it into local languages or make adaptations to suit local circumstances and conditions. The guide is not exhaustive, however; it does not cover interventions for every situation, nor are the descriptions of interventions detailed. Instead, it is designed to provide information to communities that will enable them to start the process of problem solving. More information about implementing programmes can be obtained from the organizations and documents listed in the annexes at the end of the guide.

1.1 What is a healthy village?

It is impossible to define precisely what is "healthy" for all communities, because this will depend on the perceptions of community members as to whether their village is a "good" place to live. However, a village or rural community can be considered healthy when rates of infectious diseases are low, when community members have access to basic services and health care that meet their needs, and when the community lives in a state of reasonable harmony. Examples of unhealthy and healthy villages are illustrated in Figures 1.1 and 1.2; however, these pictures show extremes and most communities will fall somewhere between the two.

1.2 Structure of the guide

The guide follows a simple format and deals with various interventions. Checklists are provided to help community leaders to assess their problems and evaluate the importance of different interventions.

An initial section looks at how good health is defined and how to identify gaps in the social and physical environment that would hinder the promotion of good health in villages. The importance of technology in improving health is then discussed, including means for providing a safe water supply and good sanitation, for safely disposing of waste and chemicals, and for providing good drainage. The importance of sustaining technologies is also emphasized, because simply installing infrastructure, such as a well or a borehole, will not improve community health if it is allowed to become nonfunctional. The importance of personal and community hygiene in promoting health is also outlined, since good hygiene practices are as important as technology for improving health.

The provision of health care and the ways in which communities can access or demand improved health care services are then discussed. This section also examines the health needs of special groups, such as pregnant women, the elderly and people with mental health problems. A final section describes the role of local governments in supporting improvements in rural health.

1.3 Using the guide and setting priorities

The guide is designed to help rural community members and health workers make informed decisions about interventions for their community health problems, by providing information about how to improve different aspects of health. Further information may be also required, such as on the detailed workings of different pit latrines, before final decisions can be made as to the best intervention. However, raising the awareness of community members about the different options for intervention should increase their participation in the decision-making process and help them to select solutions that are appropriate for their community. Although this guide provides a framework for decision-making and should help rural communities to improve the

Figure 1.1 *Unhealthy village practices*

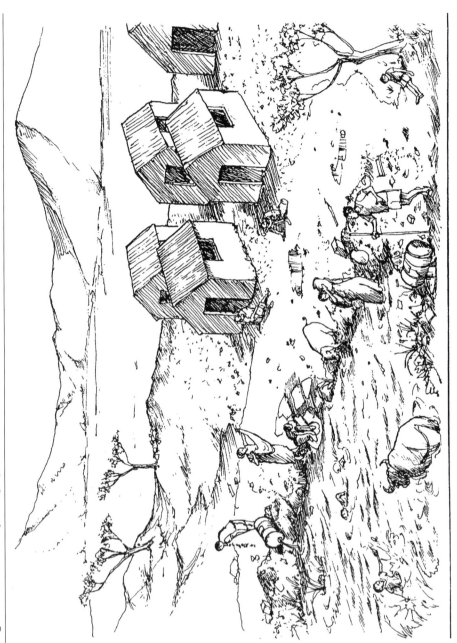

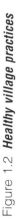

Figure 1.2 *Healthy village practices*

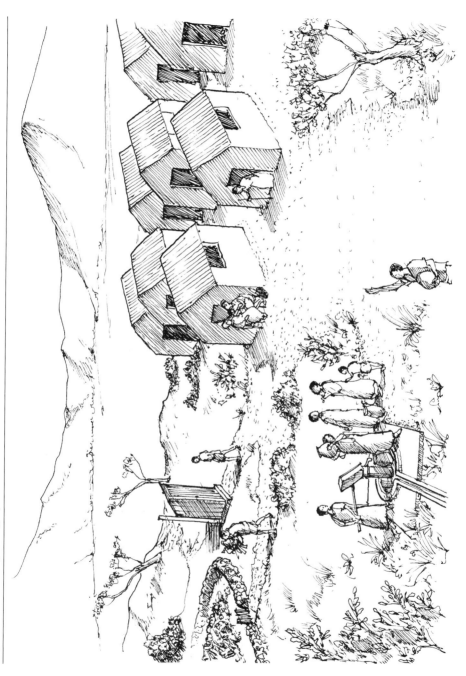

health and well-being of community members, it does not replace local professionals, who will have a more detailed understanding and knowledge of the communities they work in. To improve community health, it may also be necessary to coordinate intervention activities with service bodies such as local governments.

When considering interventions, it is important to bear in mind the current conditions in a community, as well as the community priorities. For example, a community may be prone to flooding, and have poor sanitation and an inadequate water supply. The community will need to determine which problems are most urgent and which can be dealt with later, and then decide on the interventions for dealing with the most pressing issues. The whole community, and not just a powerful few, should be involved in this decision-making process. Women, in particular, should be given a proper say in improving their village, as they may be most affected by the health problems caused by an unhealthy environment. Whenever possible, a number of interventions should be undertaken at the same time, since this may resolve health problems more quickly and cost-effectively. However, realizing these goals may require a substantial commitment of time and resources from the community, so a balance must be struck between working to improve the village environment and the needs of families to grow food and earn incomes.

CHAPTER 2

Achieving good health

According to the World Health Organization (WHO) good health is not merely the absence of disease; it is also a reflection of the social and mental well-being of people in a community. Thus, to achieve the WHO goal of providing health for all, improvements in a community should aim not simply to reduce disease, but also to reduce social tensions and mental ill-health to acceptable levels.

2.1 Factors that influence health

Many factors influence health and some may have both good and bad influences. For example, surface water bodies can be beneficial as they can supply water for domestic and agricultural work, may be used for fishing and recreation, and can create a pleasant environment. However, they can also be breeding areas for insects and snails that transmit diseases such as malaria, dengue fever and schistosomiasis. Pollution of water bodies by humans also increases the risks to health. Factors that influence health can be grouped as follows:

- The environment.
- The awareness of individuals and communities about health.
- Personal hygiene.
- Health care.
- Disease.

The linkages between these factors and health are discussed more fully below (see also Figure 2.1).

2.1.1 Environment

The environment includes both the physical environment we live in and the social fabric of the community, and both significantly influence health. The physical environment plays an important role in many ways. A clean

Figure 2.1 *Linkages between factors that affect health*

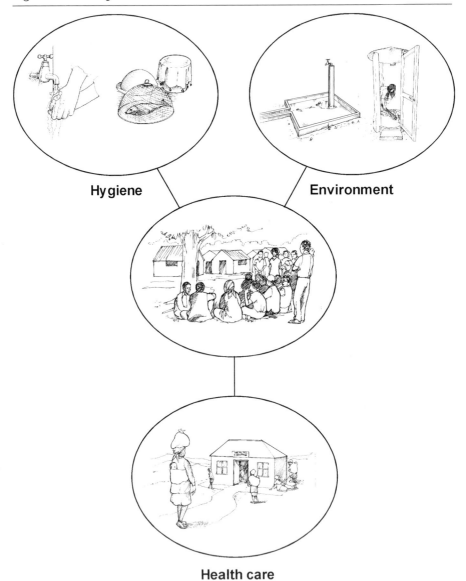

Hygiene   **Environment**

Health care

environment helps prevent the spread of disease and may reduce depression. For example, safe and adequate water supplies, sanitation, drainage and solid waste disposal all benefit health by removing disease vectors from human contact. Dirty environments, by contrast, encourage the spread of disease and may adversely influence the mental and emotional well-being of individuals.

Industry and traffic also adversely affect health by polluting the air, water and soil, and by causing accidents.

Equally important are the home and social environments. When the home environment is dirty, disease may still spread even if the rest of the village is clean; and where houses are of poor quality, with poor ventilation and lighting, other health problems may result, such as premature eyesight failure or respiratory diseases. The social environment also has a major impact on health. If people are marginalized because of gender, income status or ethnic/religious affiliation, they are more likely to be prone to anxiety and depression and to suffer mental ill-health. In particular, the status of women in the community is important. In communities where women are discriminated against, they are more likely to suffer both physical and mental ill-health. By contrast, in communities that are harmonious, accept differences and promote resolution of conflict through dialogue, the people are usually more healthy.

2.1.2 Awareness of health issues

The awareness of individuals about health is fundamental to promoting a healthier village. If people do not understand the causes of ill-health and how they can improve their health they cannot make decisions about investing resources and time to improve their village, or about lobbying for outside assistance. Such awareness should be developed in all areas that influence health because the different influences are often interrelated. Unless people accept that they need an improved environment, better personal hygiene and better access to adequate health care, investments aimed at improving health may have only limited impact. It is also essential that community members are aware that improvements in their environment or hygiene need to be sustained to achieve long-term improvements in their health. Both community leaders and governments play important roles in developing this awareness.

2.1.3 Personal hygiene

Personal hygiene is essential both for improving health and for sustaining the benefits of interventions. For example, if injuries and minor cuts are not kept clean, they may become infected and lead to further health problems. And even though water supplies and sanitation facilities may be constructed in a community, unless people use these facilities properly and wash their hands after defecation, store water safely, bathe, and clean clothes and utensils properly, diseases caused by poor water and sanitation may still exist.

2.1.4 Health care

All people suffer from disease at some point in their lives and may need to seek medical advice and treatment. Small children in particular may be prone to illnesses that require treatment and there are several infectious diseases for which immunization is recommended (which should be carried out or supervised by trained medical staff). In all cases, the health outcomes are profoundly affected by whether health care facilities are available to the people. Community leaders should therefore lobby national and regional service providers to locate health care facilities as close to communities as possible and preferably within the community itself.

2.1.5 Faecal–oral diseases

Many diseases are caused by food, water and hands that are contaminated by disease-causing organisms or "pathogens" that come from faeces. The diseases caused by these pathogens are called faecal–oral diseases because faecal material is ingested. These diseases, which include dysentery, cholera, giardiasis, typhoid and intestinal worm infections, are responsible for much sickness and many deaths each year. Many of these illnesses and deaths occur unnecessarily, since the faecal–oral routes of disease transmission are among the most easily blocked. There are several faecal–oral routes of transmission (Figure 2.2). For example, many infectious diseases are spread through poorly prepared and stored food, and many epidemics start with the consumption of poor quality food, or from drinking contaminated water. Good quality drinking-water and good personal hygiene in food preparation and handling are therefore of utmost importance in preventing the spread of these diseases.

2.1.6 Vector-borne diseases

Diseases transmitted by vectors such as mosquitoes (malaria) and sandflies (leishmaniasis) and those with intermediate hosts in fresh water such as snails (schistosomiasis) place a heavy burden on rural communities in the tropics and subtropics. They are closely linked to the characteristics of the local ecology (e.g. standing water or irrigation systems), human behaviour (water contact patterns) and socioeconomic status (capacity to maintain a clean environment). Since the flight range of most disease-carrying insects is relatively limited and the transmission of schistosomiasis is restricted to water contact points, communities can make substantial contributions towards making villages healthier by managing their environment; by using simple vector control procedures; and by cleaning the village and its surroundings. In many

Figure 2.2 *Faecal–oral routes of disease transmission*

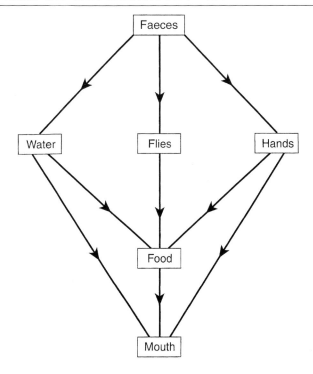

instances these procedures can be incorporated into daily village routines, for example by modifying agricultural practices.

2.2 Identifying health problems and establishing priorities

To improve the health of people in a community a number of problems may need to be resolved. While it is better to address these problems in an integrated way, it may be necessary to establish priorities and deal with the most pressing issues immediately. This situation could arise, for example, if communities or service providers have limited resources and can tackle only a few problems at a time. Community members may also have different perceptions of the main problems: people living in low-lying areas prone to flooding may feel that drainage is the major problem to be resolved, whereas those living in higher areas may be more concerned with water supply. If external bodies alone are responsible for prioritizing the issues, the priorities may not reflect community concerns and there may be a more limited sense of community ownership of a project.

Two questionnaires are provided in this guide that allow community members to identify major health issues in their community and establish health priorities. However, to ensure that community priorities are understood and that needs are met, it is essential to involve the different stakeholders in a community. Women and men, rich and poor, children and the elderly, and different ethnic and religious groups may all have different health priorities, and while it may not be possible to accommodate every view, the final list of priorities should reflect what most people believe are important health issues. To identify health problems in a community, community members should try to answer the questions listed below and then discuss the most pressing issues. During the discussion community members can try to list (or rank) the problems identified in order of importance.

Identifying community health issues

- Is diarrhoea common among children?
- Are worm infections common?
- Are respiratory (breathing) problems common?
- Are eyesight problems common, particularly among women?
- Are malaria or other vector-borne diseases common?
- Do many people have fevers?
- Have there been recent outbreaks of disease that affected many people in your community?
- Are children undernourished? Do they look thin or lack energy?
- Are there health workers or facilities (clinics or health centres) in the community?
- Do any children or adults have a mental health problem (e.g. psychosis)?
- What are the major health problems identified by community members? List them in order of importance.

2.2.1 Assessing community perceptions about health

To help identify the most important health problems in a community, the perceptions of community members about health should be assessed. It is important that all sections of the community are involved in these assessments. Different methods for achieving this goal are discussed below.

Questionnaires

One way to find out what people think is to use a community questionnaire. Because questionnaires may be answered by many people (sometimes, every household in the community) they can provide good information about the perceptions of community members towards health problems and health priorities. However, questionnaires have limitations. Frequently, it may be difficult for community members to devise their own questionnaires and the information collected may require sophisticated analysis. As a result, it is likely that nongovernmental organizations (NGOs) or local government staff will administer the questionnaires, rather than community members. Nevertheless, the community should always ask for feedback on the findings. Because the questions must be defined before the information is collected, the information will be limited to these issues. Questionnaires may not therefore be flexible enough to include other issues of importance to the community.

Participatory approaches

Because of the limitations of questionnaires, a number of other techniques have been developed. They are often grouped together and referred to as a participatory rural (or rapid) appraisal. The techniques allow the community itself to develop areas for discussion, rather than using questionnaire responses to define the topics. These techniques are sometimes used with questionnaires: by asking the same question in different ways during community discussions, issues raised by questionnaire respondents can be verified. More information about the techniques can be found in the documents listed in Annex 2. They are briefly discussed below to provide an idea of how such techniques may be used.

Participatory approaches cover a range of techniques, including key informant interviews, group discussions and observations. Although these techniques are often used by trained staff, they can also be used by community leaders to assess the perceptions of community members about health issues. When using these techniques it is important to balance the need to discuss all issues of community concern with the need to remain focused on the principal objective—assessment of community health priorities.

Key informant interviews are discussions with key people within a community who have a special interest in, or responsibility for, improving health. Key informants include women's leaders, youth leaders, religious leaders and health workers. The interviews are usually structured, in that the interviewer has the objective of obtaining information on key health issues. Rather than directly asking prepared questions, however, the interviewer can instead prepare topic guides to ensure that the principal areas of interest are covered during the course of discussions. The objective of each interview should be clearly defined and the community members best placed to provide answers should be identified.

Example topic guide
Uganda: focus group discussion on water usage

Goal:
To determine which sources of water are used for consumption.

Topics:
• What water sources are available to the community?

• Which local water sources do people commonly use?

• What are the water sources used for?

• What influences decisions to use the sources?

A focus group discussion is a technique that brings together groups of people to discuss a particular issue, often in an informal setting as illustrated in Figures 2.3 and 2.4. The role of the group facilitator is to help the group to identify key issues related to the topic under discussion, while allowing sufficient flexibility to cover all aspects of the topic to everyone's satisfaction. To help foster agreement about the key issues, it is better to establish a goal or objective that the whole group agrees with from the outset. For example, the goal may be to decide which problems are most important to resolve. Sometimes people may give responses that are not relevant, or that appear silly or amusing to the other group members. It is important that people do not feel they are being ridiculed for their views. This can be accomplished by saying, for example, "That is a good point, but maybe we need to discuss the relevance of this."

Problems may arise during group discussions which can lead to biased answers or dissatisfaction among group members. For example, the discussion may be dominated by a few individuals who express their point of view forcefully and prevent others from fully participating. Lack of contribution by some members may also be a problem and it may be necessary to directly ask such individuals what they think about a particular issue. However, care should be taken not to appear too aggressive or insistent since some people find it hard to talk in front of others. One approach that may help everyone to feel comfortable during discussion is to select individuals from specific groups, such as women or young people, rather than include a mix of people in the discussion. To overcome problems in group discussions, it is important to set ground rules at the outset of the discussion which all members agree to abide by. If this is not done, the discussion may become heated, some people may dominate the group and others may feel disappointed with the discussion.

Figure 2.3 **Focus group discussions**

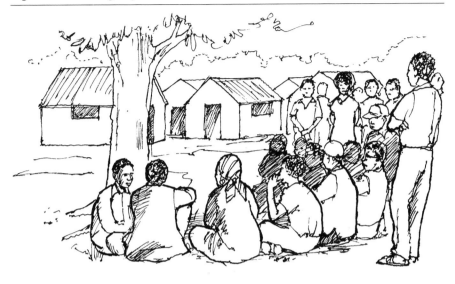

Figure 2.4 **Small community discussions**

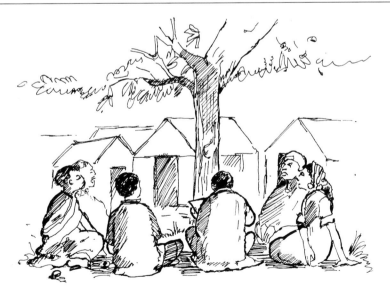

Ground rules for focus group discussions

- There are no right or wrong answers, just different opinions.

- Everyone has the right to express their opinion and should not be penalized if the group feels the opinion is not relevant or interesting.

- Only one person at a time should talk; when someone wants to contribute they should raise their hand.

- No one person should dominate the discussion—all should be allowed to contribute.

Different sections of the community may have different opinions about which problems are most important. To reflect this, different groups in the community can prepare a map that locates the most important problems. The map can then be used as a discussion tool with the groups to help community members decide which activities should be undertaken to improve the health of the overall community.

Key points for collecting information from a community

- All sections of the community should have input into the process. Priorities established by only a few people may not cover all needs adequately.

- Decide from the start how the information will be used. This should be developed with the whole community.

- Make sure the information is reliable.

2.2.2 Identifying causes of health problems

Once the major health problems in a community have been identified, the underlying causes need to be examined so that priorities for action can be ranked. For example, diarrhoea in a community may be caused by poor-quality water, by unhygienic food, or by a lack of sanitation, and the type of intervention required will depend on the nature of the underlying cause. To help identify the principal causes of ill-health in a community and the most important areas to improve, community members can complete the following questionnaire and discuss the findings with the whole community.

Identifying causes of community health problems

- What types of water supply does the community have?
- Is the water source protected and/or treated?
- How much water is collected by households?
- Is the water always available?
- Does everyone have access to water?
- Does the community know the quality of the water?
- Are there special places for bathing and laundry?
- Do households have some form of sanitation?
- What types of sanitation are there?
- Are there separate facilities for women (in areas where mixed facilities are unacceptable)?
- Is solid waste disposed of, or does waste build up in the village?
- How is solid waste disposed of?
- Are there stagnant or standing bodies of water in the community?
- Is there a system of drainage in homes and for the community?
- Is there a market in the community?
- Is the market area cleaned every day?
- Is the market dirty?
- Is meat sold at the market?
- Is the meat always fresh?
- Are market vendors careful with personal hygiene and do they keep their hands clean?
- Does the market have water supply and sanitation facilities?
- Are chemicals used or stored in the community?
- How are they stored?
- How are chemicals disposed of?
- Do houses in the community have many windows?
- What cooking fuel is used in the community?
- Where do people cook in the community?
- What materials are used for house construction?
- Are mosquitoes, flies and other insects common in the community?
- Are rats and other vermin common?
- Are cattle or other domestic animals kept close to homes?
- Are the same bodies of water used for washing, laundering and receiving human and animal wastes?

What are the major problems? List them in order of importance to the community.

2.3 **Using the information**

Whichever techniques are used it is essential that the information obtained reflects broad opinion in the community, is reliable and can be translated into action. Once the major causes of ill-health have been identified by the community and the necessary interventions agreed upon, the resources required must be identified. If the community lacks the necessary resources, representatives of the local government and NGOs can be contacted to discuss how best to carry out the improvements. It may be possible to prepare a proposal that identifies the work the community would like to undertake, how much the improvements would cost and the contributions community members themselves can make.

The time and money required to keep improved facilities working should also be considered, because benefits may be short-lived if the community cannot afford to maintain improvements. It is important therefore to discuss with community members, local governments and NGOs the long-term requirements of improvements and whether they are affordable. This will help community members to select options most suited to community needs and resources.

CHAPTER 3

Water

Water is critical to life, but it is also a limited resource and several interrelated factors are decreasing its availability. These factors include climate changes, increasing demand, lowered water tables and environmental degradation. There is also the growing threat of international and intercommunity disputes over water supplies. It is important, therefore, that communities manage their water resources better and supply water for specific uses.

For most people, it is not a problem to obtain the minimum amount of water necessary to sustain life. Rather, problems relate to the quantities of water required for different activities (resource allocation) and the quality of the water available (source suitability). Many places with water shortages actually receive abundant rainfall and community-based initiatives could alleviate water scarcity. Such initiatives may incorporate traditional approaches and include water management and conservation measures; sustainable rates of extraction; sustainable crop production; catchment protection; rainwater harvesting; and soil conservation.

3.1 Providing community water supplies

To promote community health an easily accessible water supply should be available that provides sufficient safe water to meet community needs. Household water needs can be estimated by questioning community members about their daily water use. If this is not possible, a minimum water need can be calculated by assuming that the average person uses 25 litres per day for drinking, cooking and personal hygiene. More water will be needed for laundry, but this may be available from other sources such as rivers or ponds. To ensure that the water is potable, either the water supply should be protected or the water should be treated before use. Low-risk water supplies for drinking and other domestic uses can be provided to communities in many ways. Often, unprotected water sources, such as springs, traditional wells and ponds, can be improved and this may be preferable to constructing completely new supplies. However, unprotected sources are open to contamination and pose a potential health risk. Community hygiene programmes should therefore promote the use of protected drinking-water sources.

Characteristics of low-risk water sources

- The water source is fully enclosed or protected (capped) and no surface water can run directly into it.

- People do not step into the water while collecting it.

- Latrines are located as far away as possible from the water source and preferably not on higher ground. If there are community concerns about this, expert advice should be sought.

- Solid waste pits, animal excreta and other pollution sources are located as far as possible from the water source.

- There is no stagnant water within 5 metres of the water source.

- If wells are used, the collection buckets are kept clean and off the ground, or a handpump is used.

When resources are limited, it may be necessary to decide whether greater emphasis should be placed on the quality of the water, or on its availability. Where sufficient safe water for all is not immediately available, intermediate steps should target the provision of larger quantities of lower-quality water. Deciding on an acceptable level of contamination is difficult and depends on the willingness of community members to pay increased costs for better water, as well as on their willingness to treat water within the home. If payment is required for water use, it must be affordable to the whole community. In any case, water with high levels of contamination, particularly with faeces, should never be used. Local health officials should be consulted about the quality of water provided and the level of health risk.

Many rural water supply programmes aim to develop water sources that can be fully managed by users, with only limited additional support from local government. While this can make a sense of community ownership more achievable, it also requires communities to make long-term commitments, such as maintenance of improved water sources, and even to contribute financially towards their construction. If this is not done, the water supply may deteriorate as shown in Figure 3.1. This means that it is important to involve communities during all stages of development of the improved water sources, from initial planning and implementation to long-term management. Community members should be actively involved in selecting the type of water supply they receive and have access to information that allows them to make informed decisions. However, discussions must be balanced and should also

Figure 3.1 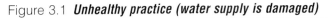 ***Unhealthy practice (water supply is damaged)***

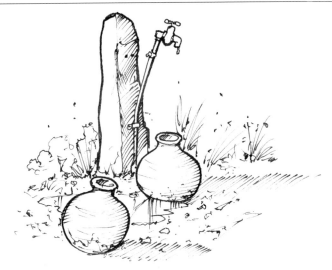

consider what the supporting agency considers feasible, not simply what the community desires. On the other hand, solutions chosen solely by outside agencies are more likely to fail.

From the outset it is also essential that community members are fully aware of the short- and long-term implications of their choices, for while it is relatively easy to build an improved water supply, sustaining it is often a major problem. For example, boreholes with handpumps are often recommended to communities, but this technology requires relatively expensive maintenance, and access to spare parts and tools is essential. In one country, spares for handpumps were available only in the capital city, a two- or three-day journey for remote communities. As a result, the handpumps were likely to fail in a very short time and the investment would have been wasted.

Checklist for communities considering water supply improvements

- Have community members been fully consulted about the type of water supply?

- Have community members had previous experiences with water supply improvements and have these been relayed to the relevant agency?

- How will the water supply be managed to ensure that it is reasonably accessible to everyone in the community?

- How will initial costs be paid and is the community expected to provide labour?

- Will labour be provided free or will the community have to raise funds to cover labour charges?

- What are the long-term financial implications of the choice of water supply?
- Can the community afford to pay expected operation and maintenance costs?
- What spare parts are required and how often should they be replaced?
- Who sells these spares and where are they obtained?
- What tools are required and where can they be obtained?
- Who will be trained to operate and maintain the water supply?
- What skills should operators have and what training will they receive?
- What long-term support can the community expect from the government and other agencies?
- If major repairs are required, whom should you contact and who will pay?
- Will the quality of the water be tested?
- How often will testing be done and how will the information be communicated to the community?

3.2 Types of water sources

3.2.1 Protected springs

A spring is where underground water flows to the surface. Springs may occur when the water table meets the ground surface; these are called gravity springs. Other times water is forced to the surface because the water-carrying layer meets an impermeable layer (gravity overflow springs or contact springs). In some cases, groundwater is held under pressure and springs come to the surface because of a natural break in the rock, or because a shallow excavation is made (artesian springs).

Springs can make very good water supplies provided that they are properly protected against contamination. If springs are found above the village, they can feed a pipe system for providing water close to homes. When a spring is at the same, or lower, level than the village, it can still be protected, but greater care is needed and it is unlikely that water will flow through the pipe system by gravity. The first step in deciding whether a spring should be protected is to determine whether it provides enough water for the expected number of users. This is easily done by measuring the time it takes for the spring to fill a bucket of known volume.

Estimating whether a water source has sufficient flow rate

- A spring fills a 20-litre bucket in 6 seconds, corresponding to a flow rate of 3.3 litres per second (20/6 = 3.3).

- In 24 hours, this spring would provide 285 000 litres (3.3 × 60 × 60 × 24).

- If each person uses 25 litres per day, the spring will supply the daily needs of 11 400 people (285 000/25).

- **NB**: a storage tank may be needed so that water flowing from the spring at night can be stored and used during the day, instead of running to waste.

To protect a spring, a retaining wall or box is constructed around the "eye" of the spring, where the water emerges from the ground. The area behind the wall or box is backfilled with sand and stones to filter water as it enters the box and help remove contamination in the groundwater. The backfill area is capped with clay and grass is planted on top.

The whole area should be fenced and a ditch dug above the spring to prevent surface water from eroding the backfill area and contaminating the spring. The collection area should be covered with concrete and sufficient space left beneath the outlet pipe for people to place jerry cans and buckets. A lined drain should be constructed to carry spilled water away from the spring. The water could be used for laundry, to feed an animal-watering trough or for irrigating a garden. In other situations spilled water may be drained to a soak-away pit or to the nearest surface water body. To prevent mosquito breeding, water from the spring should not be allowed to form pools. An example of a well-protected spring is shown in Figure 3.2.

As discussed earlier, all water supplies need to be maintained. Although protected springs require very little maintenance, far less than a borehole with handpump, the following basic checks should be carried out every 1–3 months.

Examples of basic checks for protected springs

- Does the water change colour after rain?

- Has a water-quality test been carried out recently?

- Did the community receive the results of the test?

- Is the area behind the retaining wall losing the grass cover?

- Does the retaining wall show signs of damage?

- Can this be repaired locally?

- Does the uphill ditch need clearing?

- Does the downhill ditch need clearing?

- Does the fence need repair?
- Does the grass behind the retaining wall need cutting?
- Do the outlets leak?

3.2.2 Dug wells

Dug wells are usually shallow wells dug by hand, although some may be quite deep, and they are often lined with bricks. However, unless artesian water is tapped, many dug wells go dry or have very little water in dry periods because it is difficult to sink wells below the water table without using more sophisticated techniques. In some arid areas, dug wells have traditionally been constructed in sandy riverbeds. Where flooding is rare, such wells can be improved to provide dry-season water sources. To protect the well from river

Figure 3.2 *Collecting water from a protected spring*

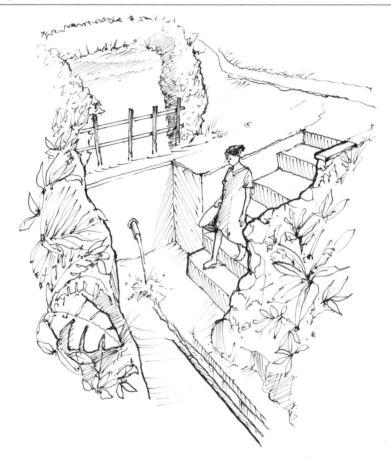

damage during the rainy seasons the well opening can be covered with a concrete slab and a concrete barrier built upstream from the well. In sandy riverbeds with water-resistant bedrock beneath, walls can be constructed under the sand to create sand dams. These collect the river water and can ensure that nearby wells are productive for longer periods in the dry season.

The shaft of an improved dug well has a concrete lining above the dry-season water table and a series of concrete rings (caissons) sunk below this level to ensure a year-round supply of water. The lining acts both to protect the shaft from collapse and to prevent surface water from infiltrating into the well at shallow depths. The top of the well (the wellhead) is built up by at least 30 cm and an apron is cast around it to prevent surface water from entering the well directly. Usually a permanent cover is put over the well and water is drawn by a handpump or windlass and bucket. People should not use their own bucket to draw water from the well as this may contaminate the water in the well. A communal rope and bucket attached to the well can be used to draw water, but the bucket and rope should be kept off the ground. One way to do this is to put a hook inside the well and always store the bucket on it. Once a dug well is completed it should be cleaned with chlorine and the pump installed.

The advantage of improved dug wells is that they can be deepened and, if the handpump or windlass fails, water can still be collected, although care should be taken not to contaminate the water by using individual buckets. However, dug wells are more likely to go dry in prolonged dry periods, or if large volumes of water are pumped from nearby deep boreholes, and they are easily contaminated. Nevertheless, they provide a low-cost water supply and communities can be actively involved in their construction. Abandoned wells should be closed to avoid polluting groundwater.

3.2.3 Boreholes

Boreholes are narrow holes drilled into the ground that tap into groundwater. Boreholes can be drilled using motorized rigs operated by trained staff, but this is expensive. Boreholes can also be drilled by hand using an augur, or by forcing water into the ground under pressure ("jetting"). If a community is involved in the actual sinking of the borehole, it is likely to use auguring or jetting because these are less expensive methods, but it is not possible to sink deep boreholes with these methods. Depending on the depth of the groundwater, a handpump may be required to bring the water to the surface. The practical limit for most handpumps is 45 metres; beyond this a motorized pump (diesel-, electric-, wind- or solar-powered) may be required.

As the borehole is drilled, a lining of plastic, steel or iron is sunk to protect the hole from collapse. The lining has slots in the bottom section to allow water to enter the borehole and gravel is placed around the bottom of the lining to improve flow and provide filtration. The top few metres around the borehole should be sealed using concrete, and a concrete apron is cast around the top of the borehole to prevent surface water from flowing into the lined shaft. A stand is usually cast into the apron to provide a stable base for the pump. Once the borehole is completed it should be cleaned with chlorine and the pump installed.

Boreholes with handpumps are often provided to villages, with the community being given responsibility for operation and maintenance. An example is shown in Figure 3.3. Unfortunately, many boreholes world-wide are no longer working because simple repairs have not been carried out. Consequently, if a borehole is drilled in a village, it is important that maintenance costs and activities can be met by the community. This may require additional training in financial management to ensure that funds can be raised for maintenance. In addition, it is particularly important to make sure that all required spares can be purchased within a reasonable distance from the village. For major repairs beyond the skills of the com-munity, clear information as to how these repairs will be carried out should be requested from the relevant agency. If the agency is unable or unwilling to provide this information, the community may not wish to commit to working with the agency, since failure of the project may not be

Figure 3.3 **Handpump on a borehole**

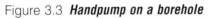

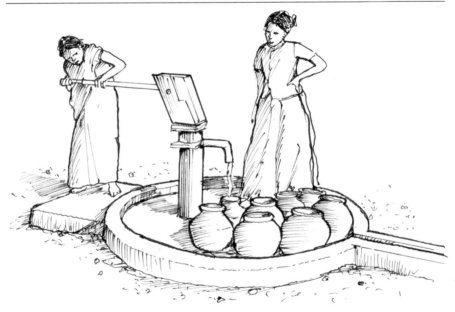

seen as the fault of the agency, and may bar the community from future support.

Boreholes usually provide good quality water, but the water sometimes contains harmful chemicals, such as fluoride and arsenic, or nuisance chemicals such as iron. Although a village would not be expected to carry out chemical analysis, community members should request that tests be carried out by the government agency or development partner, and the results fully discussed with the community. In villages with existing boreholes, community members should share their experiences with agency representatives before more boreholes are drilled. This will help both parties to make better decisions about the water supply.

Factors to consider when selecting a borehole water supply

- What training will be provided for maintaining the pump?
- What tools and materials are required for maintenance?
- What tools and materials are provided by the outside agency?
- What tools and materials must be purchased by the community?
- How much do these tools and materials cost?
- Where can spare parts be purchased?
- How much do spare parts cost?
- How often do spares need to be purchased and what is their shelf-life?

3.2.4 Piped water supply

Many villages may have piped water systems that supply communal taps or yard taps. These piped water systems are often small and rely on community management, and many use untreated groundwater sources. Small piped water systems are usually fed by gravity, either from protected springs or from surface water above the village, although some may be supplied from boreholes fitted with motorized pumps. Most piped water supplies include storage tanks so that water is always available, even when demand is heaviest. Such tanks are usually necessary because the rate of water use at peak times of the day (often early morning and early evening) is greater than the average rate of use throughout the day. The tanks also provide emergency storage in the event of a breakdown. When planning a piped system, community members should consider carefully where to locate the taps, so that everyone has relatively easy access. However, the design of piped systems can be quite complicated and it may not be possible to place taps where people would prefer.

Figure 3.4 *Single standpost with surround*

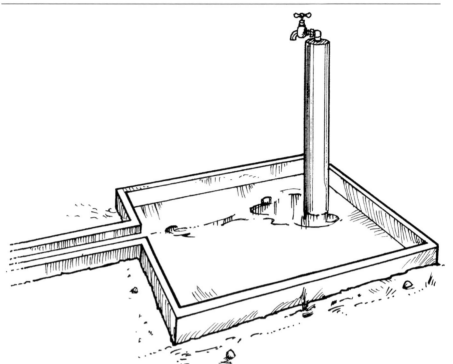

As with boreholes and handpumps, piped systems require regular maintenance. Pipe leaks need to be repaired rapidly to prevent water loss, and to prevent surface water from entering the pipes and contaminating the supply. Also, communal taps are likely to be used heavily and users may not be as careful as they would with their own taps. As a result, the taps are more likely to break and will need frequent replacement. One way of dealing with these issues is to give someone in the community responsibility for checking communal taps and making repairs. To prevent the accumulation of stagnant water around community taps, which could become mosquito breeding sites, community members could build a concrete "apron" at the base of the taps and include a drain and a soakage pit. An example of a standpost is shown in Figure 3.4.

Another problem with piped systems is that users do not consider the impact of how much water they use, and may not think it is important to turn off the tap after use. When there is a lot of water, this may not have negative consequences. However, where the amount of water available is limited, if users at the high end of the system leave taps running, users lower down may suffer shortages or intermittent service. This can force them to use less safe sources of water. Moreover, if the pipes are dry or have very low flow rates, surface water may enter the pipes and contaminate the piped water. Users of piped water systems should thus be aware of the impact of their water use on others and good water use should be promoted. This could be supported through village regulations or by-laws that penalize people who persistently abuse the system.

3.2.5 Rainwater harvesting

Although rainwater can be a good source of water for drinking and domestic use, it may be seasonal, and it is often difficult for a community to rely on rainwater alone. Collecting sufficient rainwater for an entire community also requires relatively large roofs and tanks, and the supply may still not be sufficient. Instead, rainwater is usually collected by households for their own use. If the rainwater is to be used for drinking it is better to collect it from a roof, rather than from a ground catchment where it may become contaminated. Ground catchments are more appropriate for agricultural use.

Using roofs to collect rainwater is relatively easy and a lot of water can be collected. For example, 50 mm of rainfall on a 4 m^2 roof yields 200 litres of water. All that is required are gutters around the roof that discharge into a collection tank. The roofing material is important and hard surfaces, such as iron sheets or tiles, allow more rain to be collected than softer surfaces such as thatch and grass, which absorb water. Hard surfaces are also easier to keep clean and are less likely to have insects and animals living in them.

Any roof used to collect rainwater for human consumption must be thoroughly cleaned at the start of the rainy period. Birds and animals may leave faeces on the roof and these can be a source of pathogens. There should be a system for diverting the flow of water in gutters away from the tank, so that the first rains (which are more likely to pick up contamination from the roof) are not collected. A small filter may be added to the top of the collection tank as an added protection. The tank should also be cleaned every year and any silt or algal matter removed. After cleaning and before use, the tank should be scrubbed using a chlorine solution (bleach).

Water should be drawn from a tap at the base of the tank, rather than with a bucket, which may contaminate the water. It is better not to bury the collection tank, even partially, since contaminated water from the soil can enter the tank. Covering the tank is also essential for preventing contamination of the water and for reducing opportunities for disease vectors to breed.

3.2.6 **Ponds, lakes and water treatment**

Ponds and lakes have traditionally been used as sources of drinking-water. Although they are easily contaminated, the water quality can be improved by careful use. For example, if platform steps or ramps are constructed at the water edge, people can be encouraged not to walk into the pond or lake when collecting water. This rapidly stops the discharge of guinea-worm eggs into the water, thus interrupting transmission. Preventing urination and defecation close to or in the pond may reduce schistosomiasis. Even so, dirt deposited on these structures can enter the pond, especially when it rains. Pumps mounted on the banks of ponds can also supply water to people away from the pond, but these may be difficult to maintain. Alternatively, a protected intake with a layer of sand as filter can be constructed in the pond or lake and be connected to a handpump. Whichever method is used, however, domestic water drawn from ponds and lakes must always be treated before consumption. Although water treatment can be complicated, communities do operate and maintain simple water-treatment plants. Some simple technologies are robust and have been community-managed in Latin America and parts of Asia. They are usually based on several filtration stages and tend not to use expensive chemicals and dosing equipment.

Pond or lake water is easily contaminated and should be treated with a disinfectant as a minimum. The most commonly used disinfectant is chlorine, although others can be used. Chlorine can be added as a solution of calcium hypochlorite, as chlorine gas or as other chlorine compounds. Achieving the correct ratio of chlorine and water is complicated, however; using too little chlorine will not kill the pathogens, while using too much will make the water taste unpleasant.

Some treatment systems, called package plants, come ready constructed. Package plants have been promoted on the basis of their low operational requirements; however, when package plants fail they usually require specialist repairs and equipment beyond the means of a small community. This should be taken into consideration when deciding whether to use a package plant.

3.3 **Household water treatment**

Sometimes the best option for improving water quality is to treat water in the home, by boiling, filtering, chlorinating or leaving the water to settle. These options are discussed in more detail in the following sections.

3.3.1 **Boiling**

Bringing water to a rolling boil will destroy pathogens in the water and make it safe to drink. Boiled water tastes "flat", but if it is left for a few hours in a partly filled, covered container, it will absorb air and lose its flat taste.

3.3.2 **Canvas filters**

Canvas bags are the simplest type of home filter. The bag is filled with water and the water collected as it seeps out of the bag. This makes the water cleaner and, although it does not remove all pathogens, is particularly useful for removing *Cyclops* containing guinea-worm eggs. Bags that have been specially treated to prevent them from rotting are available.

3.3.3 **Candle filters**

Candle filters are hollow, porous ceramic cartridges. Although they do not filter out all pathogens, they should remove the larger ones such as protozoa, worms and bacteria (but not viruses). Ceramic candles need careful maintenance and should be cleaned and boiled at least once a week, even if they are not clogged. If a candle filter becomes clogged, it should be scrubbed under running water with a stiff brush free of soap, grease or oil. To reduce the risk that water will pass through a candle without being filtered, such as through a small crack, candle filters should be regularly inspected and replaced if necessary. In some countries it is common to both filter and boil water. Where this is done, the water should be filtered first and then boiled. Some filters incorporate silver into the candle, but this does not disinfect the water and the candle acts simply as a normal filter.

3.3.4 **Disinfection**

One method of treating water in households is to add chlorine. This will kill most bacteria and some viruses. Since the taste of chlorine disappears when water is left in open containers, a very small lump of bleaching powder or one drop of household bleach can be added to a 20-litre water container and the mix left to stand for at least 30 minutes. After this time, if a faint smell of chlorine can be detected in the water, it should be low-risk and palatable to drink. Chlorine should only be added to clear water otherwise it will be absorbed by the dirt in the water. Moreover, chlorine that has been stored for some time will lose potency. The use of disinfectants as a household treatment system has been successfully implemented in Latin America and Asia.

Other disinfection systems have been developed for treating household water, particularly the use of solar radiation. There are some simple methods of solar disinfection (e.g. SODIS), which can effectively treat water, although this may take longer than chlorine disinfection.

Household water treatment

In Bolivia, household water treatment was introduced into two communities where water quality was generally poor. The treatment used mixed oxidants (including chlorine) and a container fitted with a tap. After the treatment was introduced, faecal contamination of water samples was reduced by over 90% and the incidence of diarrhoea dropped by almost 50%. Similar improvements have been observed in other countries, such as Bangladesh, demonstrating that household treatments can be effective.

Source: Quick RE et al. Diarrhoea prevention in Bolivia through point-of-use water treatment and safe storage: a promising new strategy. *Epidemiology and Infection*, 1999 122:83–90.

3.3.5 Settling

Where water is cloudy or muddy, a simple treatment is to allow particulates in the water to settle overnight. Clear water at the top of the container is then poured into a clean container. Adding certain chemicals can help settling, such as a pinch of aluminium sulfate (alum), or powder from the ground seeds of *Moringa oleifera* (horseradish tree) and *Moringa stenopetala*, sprinkled onto the water surface.

It should be stressed that settling does NOT remove all pathogens, silt or clay. The settling of particles may reduce pathogens but some will remain, and water should be boiled or disinfected before it is consumed.

3.4 Safe handling of water

Frequently, water collected from a communal point and transported back to houses for use becomes contaminated because of poor handling. Community members should therefore be aware of the risks of contaminating the water and how it can be prevented.

All water containers should be clean, especially inside. It is always best to clean the insides of storage containers with either detergent or chlorine. Leaving a capful of bleach in a sealed plastic or metal container full of water for 30 minutes will kill most pathogens. If detergent or chlorine is not available, the insides of clay pots can be cleaned with ash. Plastic or metal containers should be cleaned weekly by putting clean sand and water inside them and shaking for a few minutes. The top of the water container should be covered to stop dust and other contaminants falling into the drinking-water. It is best for water to be poured from the container to prevent contact with dirty fingers and hands. An example of a good storage container is shown in Figure 3.5.

When scoops are used to take water out of the storage container they should be clean and kept inside the water storage jar. They should never be placed on the floor.

3.5 **Monitoring water quality**

Water of poor microbial quality can have a significant impact on the health of community members by causing disease and contributing to the spread of epidemics. Water quality should therefore be monitored on a regular basis. Ideally, it should be tested by staff working with local and national government in support of the Healthy Villages programme. The community should request that such support is given by the local authorities, particularly if it suspected that the community water supply is contaminated. The test results should be provided to the community and if any problems arise, the community should request recommendations for solutions.

3.5.1 **Microbial quality**

The major concern of microbiological testing is whether faeces have contaminated the water supply, as most of the infectious water-related diseases, such as cholera and dysentery, are caused by faecal contamination. Although these diseases can also be transmitted through poor hygiene and inadequate

Figure 3.5 *Household storage container*

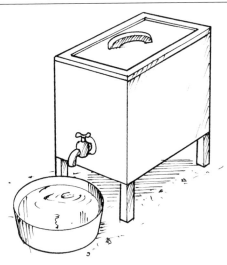

sanitation, control of drinking-water quality is one of the main ways of preventing their spread.

Using surveillance to promote better management of water quality

Environmental health staff from local councils in Uganda used water quality tests as a way of working with communities to identify problems. The staff took water samples from sources and households, and then left the water testing kit overnight so that community members could perform the tests themselves. The next day the results were discussed with community members. The discussions were always lively and the approach helped to improve both the management of protected springs and water handling and hygiene practices. Discussing the results of water quality tests with communities was an effective way of promoting improvements.

The principal method of assessing the microbial quality of water is to test for bacteria whose presence indicates that faeces may be in the water. An analysis of the test results is usually beyond the resources of communities and will be carried out by health or water officials. However, community members can request that officials regularly test the water supply and inform the community of the results and recommendations. Some kits have been developed for community use, but the results of these tests should be analysed with caution.

3.5.2 Sanitary inspection

An analysis of water quality usually also includes a sanitary inspection. This is a visual assessment of the water supply, using standard forms to record information, to see whether faecal pollution exists and whether such pollution could reach the water source. Sanitary inspections can be undertaken by communities on a regular basis as part of operation and maintenance, and forms have been developed in several countries to help communities undertake these inspections. Many of the risks to the water supply relate to improper operation and maintenance activities in the area around the water source, and sanitary inspection can be used to ensure that these tasks are carried out to keep the water supplies safe. Examples of sanitary inspection forms for community use are available in a number of the documents listed in Annex 2.

3.5.3 Chemical quality

It may also be necessary to test community water supplies for harmful chemicals. Certain chemicals, such as fluoride, nitrate and arsenic, represent a health risk, whereas others, for example iron, manganese and sulfate, may cause consumers to reject the water because it is unpleasant to drink or stains clothes and causes other problems. Testing is usually done by health or water officials, but community members can play a key role by demanding that such analyses are carried out, and by informing officials of any developments that may cause contamination of the water supply. When a water supply is first developed, a full water quality analysis should be carried out. The community should request feedback regarding this analysis and ask for guidance concerning the suitability of the water source for drinking.

3.6 Managing community water resources

Communities need to conserve water resources for future generations; ways in which this can be accomplished are discussed in the following sections.

3.6.1 Preventing over-pumping of groundwater

Communities should discuss with outside agencies the short- and long-term impacts of water supply improvement on water resources. For example, sinking too many tubewells for irrigation may cause serious depletion of water held underground and even cause water sources to dry up. This can also lead to deteriorating water quality: as the water table falls, domestic tubewells must be sunk deeper into underground water that may contain harmful chemicals such as fluoride or arsenic. Because community members are the principal stakeholders of local water resources, they should always ask planning agencies to assess the longer-term effects of water pumping on the environment and should be actively involved in evaluating the risks.

3.6.2 Water conservation

Although it is important that people use enough water for good hygiene, in areas where water is scarce it is also important not to waste water. Piped water supplies are particularly vulnerable to wastage; if they are not properly managed, the community as a whole may suffer water shortages and people will have to wait longer to collect water. Most piped water systems leak and need to be checked regularly and repaired as soon as faults are discovered. Taps should also be turned off immediately after use and children discouraged from playing with taps.

Questions to ask in areas prone to water shortages

- Does the main water source dry up?
- If so, where will water be collected?

- How far away are alternative sources of water and how long does it take to collect the water?
- Who collects the water and how often do they have to go to the source?
- How much water do families collect each day?
- Does the source provide sufficient water?
- Are there problems with water quality?
- Would rain failure next season bring a drought?
- What would be the effect on pasture, vegetation and crops?
- What would be the traditional response to drought?

3.6.3 Managing water for agriculture

Farmers can protect their lands by building small stone dykes or growing hedges along the edges of fields. These prevent rainwater from running down slopes too fast and reduce erosion. Some of the rainwater infiltrates the soil, and crops near the dykes have a higher survival rate in times of water stress and produce yields about 40% higher than crops further from the dykes. The amount of water that goes into the groundwater is also higher in these areas.

The introduction or expansion of irrigated agriculture will cause important changes in the local hydrology, land use patterns and ecology. Such changes may introduce new health risks into the area, although there are ways to manage these risks. Some examples of health risks and how they may be managed are listed below.

- When irrigation is permanently introduced into arid areas, habitats for disease vectors, such as the malaria-carrying anopheline mosquitoes, can also be created. This is particularly a problem in low-lying areas where drainage is poor and pools of stagnant water appear. Also, if the local drinking-water wells become saline, the community may use irrigation channels as a source of drinking-water, increasing the risk of diarrhoeal disease, of schistosomiasis (from contact with the water) and of exposure to agrochemical residues. To help counter these risks, the community can take measures such as maintaining proper drainage, ensuring water systems are well-maintained and filling ground depressions.
- Water storage facilities are an essential part of many irrigation systems, but small dams/reservoirs and tanks can pose health risks by acting as breeding habitats for disease vectors, and as foci for transmitting schistosomiasis and guinea-worm infections. Options for a Healthy Village approach include fencing off reservoirs, varying the water reservoir levels, removing weeds and flushing the surrounding areas.
- Mosquitoes often breed in areas flooded for rice production, but the

breeding cycle can be interrupted by alternately flooding and drying the rice plots (as opposed to continuous flooding). A well-designed regime will also save water and may even increase rice yield.

- Irrigation water demands can be reduced by recycling treated wastewater. Recycled wastewater can be used productively to irrigate fruit, such as papaya and banana, or for irrigating vegetable gardens. Eucalyptus and papyrus should be avoided, since they are "water-hungry" plants. Safe use of wastewater is discussed further in section 4.2.

CHAPTER 4

Excreta disposal

Safe disposal of excreta, so that it does not contaminate the environment, water, food or hands, is essential for ensuring a healthy environment and for protecting personal health. This can be accomplished in many ways, some requiring water, others requiring little or none. Regardless of method, the safe disposal of human faeces is one of the principal ways of breaking the faecal–oral disease transmission cycle. Sanitation is therefore a critical barrier to disease transmission.

Plans for locating sanitation facilities, and for treating and removing waste, must consider cultural issues, particularly as sanitation is usually focused on the household. Excreta disposal may be a difficult subject for a community to discuss: it may be taboo, or people may not like to discuss issues they regard as personal and unclean. In some cases, people may feel that sanitation facilities are not appropriate for children, or that children's faeces are not harmful. In others, separate facilities may be required for men and women, and it may be necessary to locate the facilities so that no one can be seen entering the latrine building. If the disposal facilities smell and are a breeding ground for flies, people may not use them.

Health improvement comes from the proper use of sanitation facilities, not simply their physical presence, and they may be abandoned if the level of service does not meet the social and cultural needs of community members at an affordable cost, as shown in Figure 4.1. Within a community, several different sanitation options may be required, with varying levels of convenience and cost (sometimes called a sanitation ladder). The advantage of this approach is that it allows households to progressively upgrade sanitation facilities over time.

4.1 Technologies for excreta disposal

Technologies for excreta disposal, with illustrations, are briefly discussed below. More detailed information is provided in the references cited in Annex 2.

Figure 4.1 *Disused latrine*

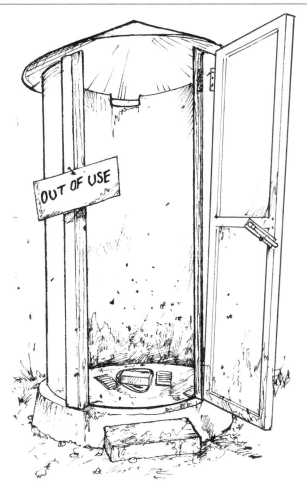

4.1.1 Cartage

Cartage is the most basic form of excreta disposal—faeces are collected in a container and disposed of daily. An example is the bucket latrine, in which household wastes are collected in buckets under a hole in the floor of a specific room. Each day, the bucket is emptied into a larger container and the contents disposed of. Bucket latrines should not be promoted because they pose health risks to both users and collectors and may spread disease. If cartage is considered for your community, a vault latrine (a latrine where wastes are stored in a sealed container) that is mechanically emptied on a regular basis is a better choice.

4.1.2 **Pit latrines**

In most pit latrine systems, faecal matter is stored in a pit and left to decompose. Unless specifically designed, pit latrines do not require periodic emptying; once a pit is full it is sealed and a new pit dug. If faecal matter is left to decompose in dry conditions for at least two years, the contents can be safely emptied manually and the pit reused. Indeed, some pit latrines are designed to allow faecal matter to compost and be reused in agriculture. Other designs use two alternating pits, reducing the need for new pits. Some pit designs are meant to be completely dry, while some use small quantities of water. Ventilation to remove odours and flies is incorporated into certain designs, while others are very basic and use traditional materials and approaches. As with all sanitation designs, it is important to know what community members want and can pay for before embarking on construction. An example of an improved pit latrine is shown in Figure 4.2.

Sanplat

The sanplat is the cheapest and most basic pit latrine. It is a small concrete platform (usually 60 cm × 60 cm or smaller), laid on top of logs or other supporting material traditionally used to cover the pit. The purpose of the sanplat is to provide a sanitary (san) platform (plat) which can be easily cleaned to limit the presence of helminths such as hookworm. Once the pit is full, the sanplat can easily be moved. However, the sanplat design does not overcome problems with odours or flies and may not be acceptable to some community members. The sanplat is best used when there is very little money for improving sanitation and where odours and flies will be tolerated.

The VIP latrine

The VIP (ventilated improved pit) latrine is designed to overcome some of the problems with traditional latrine designs, but it is more expensive than a sanplat. It has a vent pipe from the pit to above the roof of the building as shown in Figures 4.3 and 4.4. When air flows across the top of the vent pipe, air is drawn up the pipe from the pit and fresh air is drawn into the pit from the building. Offensive odours from the pit thus pass through the vent pipe and do not enter the building. The location of VIP latrines is important: unless a clear flow of air is maintained across the top of the vent, the ventilation system may not be effective. VIP latrines should therefore be located away from trees or high buildings that may limit airflow. A dark vent pipe also helps the air to rise. The top of the pipe is usually covered with mosquito meshing. If the inside of the building is kept partially dark, the flies will be attracted to light at the top of the pipe, where they will be trapped and die.

Figure 4.2 *Improved pit latrine*

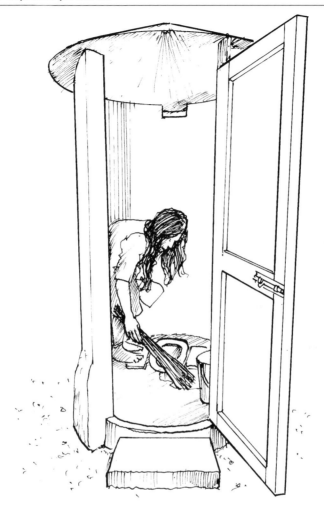

When the VIP latrine is constructed and used properly, it provides great improvements in fly and odour control, but may not eliminate either completely.

A VIP latrine is designed to work as a dry system, with any liquid in the content infiltrating into the surrounding soil. Although some liquid inevitably will enter the pit, it should be minimized. For example, it would not be appropriate to dispose of household wastewater into the pit as this may prevent decomposition of the contents. VIP latrines are most appropriate where people do not use water for cleaning themselves after defecating, but use solid materials such as paper, corncobs or leaves.

Figure 4.3 **Twin pit latrine**

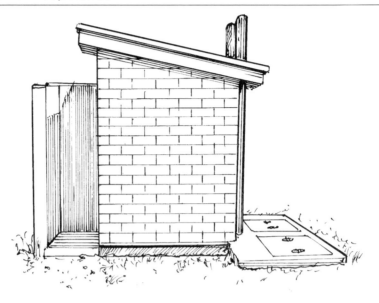

Figure 4.4 **VIP latrine**

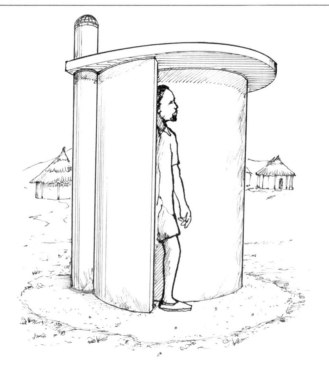

VIP latrines may be designed with single or double pits. Double pits may be used, for example, when cultural taboos prohibit the mixing of male and female faeces. Twin pits may also be used to facilitate emptying and composting. When one pit is full, the other can be emptied and reused. The pit of a VIP latrine is usually located directly beneath the slab to prevent fouling of the chute, which would lead to odour and fly problems, and require regular cleaning.

The VIP latrine is more expensive than either traditional designs or the sanplat and this should be borne in mind when considering its use. In some areas, traditional latrines or sanplat latrines can be improved by providing ventilation. However, it likely that traditional floor materials will allow light to enter the pit, which will make fly control more difficult. Installing a vent pipe on an existing latrine may damage it. When considering a VIP latrine as an improvement on existing sanitation, it is important to be aware that this may require the construction of a new latrine, not simply the upgrading of an existing one.

Pour–flush latrines

A pour–flush latrine is a type of pit latrine where small volumes of water (commonly 1–3 litres) are used to flush faeces into the pit. They are most appropriate where people use water to clean themselves after defecating (e.g. in Muslim cultures) and where people have access to reliable water supplies close to the home. Solid materials should not be disposed of into pour–flush latrines, as this could block the pipe and even cause it to break.

A pour–flush latrine has a small collection pan set in a slab. Wastes are disposed of through a section of pipe bent into a U shape (a U-bend) to maintain a water seal for reducing fly and odour problems. A vent pipe may also be added to the pit to help with fly and odour problems. The pit of a pour–flush latrine may be located directly beneath the slab or set to one side, but offset pits may require more water to prevent blockages. The pit is usually connected to a soakaway to allow liquids to infiltrate the soil, leaving solid waste to decompose. Pour–flush latrines can also be designed to be connected to small-bore sewers at a later date. As with VIP latrines, twin pits may be used.

4.1.3 Septic tanks

A septic tank is a form of on-site sanitation that provides the convenience of a sewerage system. It is usually linked to flush toilets and can receive domestic wastewater (or sullage). Since flush toilets tend to use large amounts of water, septic tanks are usually appropriate only for households with water piped into the home. The tank is offset from the house and linked to the toilet and domestic wastewater by a short drain. It is designed to hold solids and is linked to a soakaway to dispose of liquid waste (effluent).

Septic tanks generally require relatively large amounts of land and periodic emptying by vacuum tankers. This is often expensive and the trucks will need easy access to the tank. Septic tanks thus tend to be high-cost solutions for improving sanitation. They are commonly used only by communities whose members have access to water supply within the home, have land available and who can afford the cost of emptying the tanks. Communal septic tanks may be feasible if a large number of households close to the tank can be connected with very short lengths of sewer pipe. For such a system to work, however, each household needs sufficient water to flush faeces into the septic tank effectively. This approach will probably be effective only when water is supplied to at least one tap on each plot.

4.1.4 Aquaprivies

An aquaprivy is similar to a septic tank; it can be connected to flush toilets and take most household wastewater. It consists of a large tank with a water seal formed by a simple down pipe into the tank to prevent odour and fly problems. Its drawback is that water must be added each day to maintain the water seal, and this is often difficult to do unless water is piped into the home. The tank is connected to a soakaway to dispose of effluent. Unlike a septic tank, the aquaprivy tank is located directly below the house, but it, too, requires periodic emptying and must be accessible to a vacuum tanker. Aquaprivies are expensive and do not offer any real advantages over pour–flush latrines.

4.1.5 Sewerage systems

Sewerage systems are designed to collect excreta and domestic wastewater and transport them away from homes to a treatment and/or disposal point. All sewerage systems require water for flushing waste away. Conventional sewerage is a high-cost sanitation option; it is usually deep-laid and must be maintained by professional staff. Such a system is thus appropriate only where funds are available for operation and maintenance by trained staff. All sewerage systems should be linked to a treatment plant, as the raw faeces they carry represent a public health risk

Modified sewerage systems are also designed to transport waste away from the home, but work on different principles from conventional sewerage systems. They do not require high-volume flush toilets, but do need significant amounts of water for flushing. At least one tap on each plot or property is therefore essential. Small-bore sewers are designed to carry only effluent, and each home requires an interceptor tank to collect and store solid material, which must be regularly emptied by mechanical means.

Shallow sewers are larger-diameter sewers that carry both solid and liquid wastes. They differ from conventional sewers in that solids deposited in the pipes are resuspended when water builds up behind the blockage. To ensure that enough water is available to move the solids, all household wastewater should be disposed of into the sewer.

While both of these modified sewerage systems have problems, they have been successfully managed by communities and have far lower water requirements than conventional sewers. The modified technologies may be appropriate in larger villages that have water supplies close to, or within, the homes.

4.2 Sewage treatment and reuse

All wastes in sewerage or septic tank systems require treatment before disposal, so that surface water and groundwater sources are not contaminated and communities are not exposed to health risks from untreated sewage. This can be accomplished either through high-cost conventional treatment systems, or through a series of waste stabilization ponds (or lagoons).

4.2.1 Stabilization ponds

Waste stabilization ponds require more land, but are cheaper and easier to operate and maintain, and need fewer trained staff than other treatment systems. The final water from waste stabilization ponds can be very good if the ponds are properly maintained. Without proper maintenance, however, the quality of the final effluent may be poor and pose a risk to health if it is used for irrigation.

In usual configurations, sewage flows through a series of ponds where the solid and liquid wastes undergo natural breakdown processes, including microbial activity. Usually, at least two ponds are used, and more commonly three. If the sludge (the solid part of the waste) from septic tanks is to be treated in a waste stabilization pond, it should go into a special pond at the start of the series because it is potentially highly toxic. Subsequent ponds treat effluent (the liquid part of the waste). Wastewater in stabilization ponds tends to have a high organic content and can serve as breeding sites for *Culex* mosquitoes that transmit lymphatic filariasis and other infections. The ponds should therefore be sited well away from human habitation, at least beyond the flying distance of the mosquitoes (over a kilometre with wind assistance).

4.2.2 **Wastewater and sludge reuse**

As society uses more water, the demand on natural water resources becomes ever greater. Some of the demands for water, particularly for agriculture and fish breeding, can be met by reusing properly treated effluent, since the water quality requirements for these purposes are not as high as for drinking-water. Treated wastewater can also be used to recharge groundwater resources, although this will be usually be undertaken as part of a national groundwater management strategy.

Benefits of reusing treated sewage effluent and sludge

- It reduces the costs of abstracting irrigation water.
- It reduces demand on valuable water resources.
- It reduces the costs to farmers of expensive inorganic fertilizers.
- It stabilizes soils, maintains good organic content, and improves the long-term productivity of the soil.
- It promotes better use of water resources.
- It decreases pollution by reducing the waste load discharged into water bodies.

The use of untreated wastewater in agriculture or aquaculture poses high health risks to farmers and consumers alike, and only the reuse of *treated* wastewater should be promoted. The treated wastes should not contain pathogens (bacteria, viruses, helminths or protozoa), because these could contaminate products and infect consumers, or be accidentally ingested by farmers during handling. Properly operated sewage-treatment plants should produce treated effluent of good enough quality for use in irrigation or fish-breeding ponds. If treated wastewater is to be reused, the community should ask the operator of the sewage-treatment plant or the local health body to carry out regular monitoring to ensure that the effluent is safe.

Solid waste from pit latrines and sewage-treatment plants can also be a valuable resource for farmers as an organic fertilizer and soil conditioner, provided that it has been allowed to properly decompose and contains no pathogens. It is particularly important to ensure that roundworm (*Ascaris*) eggs are no longer infective. Normally, it takes two years for the waste in a pit latrine to decompose, but longer if the pit is wet. Some composting pit latrines (e.g. the Viet Nam latrine) accelerate the decomposition of sludge and inactivation of roundworm eggs by increasing the temperature in the sludge pile. Before your community reuses sludge, however, health officials should be consulted about the minimum time for sludge decomposition. If possible, the quality of the sludge should occasionally be tested. However, testing for microorganisms such as protozoa and helminths is expensive, and it may be more effective to use retention time to judge whether the sludge will be safe to use.

While the microbial quality of treated effluent and sludge is the major health concern, chemical contamination is also a consideration. In particular, wastewater reuse may increase the nitrate and chloride content of the soil. Nitrate has been linked to the "blue-baby" syndrome that can be fatal in infants. Although chloride is not a health concern, it can increase water salinity and affect soil fertility. If community members suspect that a water source is contaminated with chemicals, they should seek the advice of local health and environment officials and request that periodic monitoring of wastewater quality be carried out.

When wastewater is reused, care should be taken to separate domestic effluent from industrial effluent, since the industrial effluent may contain chemicals harmful to health or the environment, such as heavy metals. If industrial sewage is mixed with domestic sewage, it is therefore not advisable to reuse the wastewater. Food products fertilized with such wastewater may pose a health risk to consumers, and the repeated application of solid or liquid wastes may cause chemical build-up in soils, leading to long-term problems for water resources.

CHAPTER 5

Drainage

5.1 Problems caused by poor drainage

Removing stormwater and household wastewater (sometimes called "sullage") is an important environmental health intervention for reducing disease. Poorly drained stormwater forms stagnant pools that provide breeding sites for disease vectors. Because of this, some diseases are more common in the wet season than the dry season. Household wastewater may also contain pathogens that can pollute groundwater sources, increasing the risk of diseases such as lymphatic filariasis. Poor drainage can lead to flooding, resulting in property loss, and people may even be forced to move to escape floodwaters. Flooding may also damage water supply infrastructure and contaminate domestic water sources.

Drainage and public health

In areas where drainage and sanitation are poor, water runs over the ground during rainstorms, picks up faeces and contaminates water sources. This contributes significantly to the spread of diseases such as typhoid and cholera, and may increase the likelihood of contracting worm infections from soil contaminated by faeces. Flooding itself may displace populations and lead to further health problems.

Source: Kolsky P. *Storm drainage: an intermediate guide to the low-cost evaluation of system performance.* London, Intermediate Technology Publications, 1998.

Drains from irrigated fields should also be properly designed and maintained, since the introduction or improvement of irrigation is often associated with an increase in the numbers of people with schistosomiasis. This is particularly true where earth drains are used and the water supply and sanitation are inadequate. Lining and properly grading the drains, removing aquatic weeds and constructing self-draining structures are all important measures for reducing health and environmental risks.

5.2 Methods for improving drainage

Designing and constructing drainage systems require expert advice from engineers to make sure that water flows away quickly and smoothly and is disposed of in a surface watercourse or soakaway. Drainage installed by one community should not create problems for other communities downstream, nor should it affect ecologically important sites. Environmental considerations should be given adequate attention: long-term changes to the environment may lead to greater health problems in the future.

5.2.1 Stormwater drains

The detailed design of stormwater drains should be carried out by engineers and take into account climatic and hydrological data. These data may be scarce, or may not cover the community where work is to be carried out. In such cases, the community can help by describing where major flood problems occur in the village and providing information about previous floods. Stormwater drains should be designed to collect water from all parts of the community and lead it to a main drain, which then discharges into a local river (Figure 5.1). The size of the drains should be calculated according to the amount of water they would be expected to carry in a storm. More extreme floods occur relatively infrequently; to provide a safety margin, the maximum

Figure 5.1 *Stormwater drain through a village*

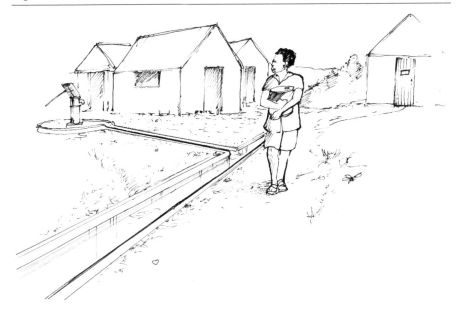

flow of water is usually calculated on the basis of floods expected to occur once every 10 or more years. If drains are designed to carry only the amount of water expected from an annual flood, they will not be able to cope with the flow of water from heavier floods, which may occur as often as every 2–3 years. This may make flooding problems worse and increase the health risks.

Stormwater drains are best constructed using a concrete lining. Earth drains are more likely to become clogged and overgrown, and cause problems with stormwater flow during minor floods. This can lead to the formation of stagnant pools and result in breeding sites for disease vectors, such as mosquitoes, increasing the risk of malaria, and snails, increasing the risk of schistosomiasis. The drains must also be properly maintained and cleaned: it is common to find that new drains become dumps for solid waste or even sewage because of inadequate maintenance. The community should therefore establish how often drains are to be cleaned and who will be responsible for the maintenance. Often, the best solution is for community members themselves to take responsibility.

Community participation in maintaining drains

It is often essential that community members participate in maintaining drains. In Indonesia, for example, residents agreed to clean the drains in front of their houses every day and this was inspected twice a week. Community members responded well to friendly inspectors who provided support for clearing the drains. Maintaining the drains soon became part of the daily routine for responsible community members.

Source: *Surface water drainage for low-income communities.* Geneva, World Health Organization, 1991

5.2.2 Sullage disposal methods

Every household generates sullage. For instance, it has been estimated that each person generates 15–20 litres per day when collecting water from a standpipe. Sullage may be disposed of either at home, using on-site methods, or through the drainage system. When sullage is disposed of at home a soakaway pit can be constructed. Alternatively, sullage can be used to irrigate small gardens, thus improving the crop yield and nutrition, and this should be promoted if possible. However, sullage can be reused this way only if it contains little or no detergent, which may damage crops.

If a soakaway is used, the pit should be located away from the house and away from water sources. Ideally, there should be a minimum of 30 metres between the soakaway pit and the nearest water source, but this distance may need to be increased if houses are uphill of water sources. It is not recommended that sullage be disposed of in pit latrines, since this may interfere with the breakdown of excreta within the pit, and may overload latrine soak-aways where pour–flush latrines are used. When the household is connected to a form of sewerage, sullage can be disposed off in the toilet or latrine. Indeed, for some sewerage systems (such as shallow sewerage or conventional sewerage) disposal of sullage in this way ensures better functioning of the system.

5.2.3 Combined drains

Combined drains are designed to carry both stormwater and sullage. Unless a combined drain is well designed and maintained, however, sullage will pool within the drain and form insect breeding sites. These problems can be overcome by using a system with a small insert drain that carries the sullage into a larger drain for carrying stormwater. As with all drainage systems, it is essential that the drains are properly operated and maintained, and that refuse is cleared from the drains.

5.2.4 Buried drains and combined sewers

Drains may also be incorporated into sewerage systems and be buried. This is more appropriate for urban areas, but can be considered in rural areas if the village roads are paved and if flood flows are significant. Buried drains have inlet chambers at regular intervals, usually along roadsides, that allow the entry of stormwater. The drains then lead directly either to a watercourse or to a sewage-treatment works. When drains flow directly into sewage-treatment works, care must be taken not to overload the works. The stormwater should always flow either into a stabilization pond, or into a storage pool constructed to take stormwater flows above a certain volume.

CHAPTER 6

Solid waste management and chemical safety

To keep the household and village environment clean and to reduce health risks, solid waste (refuse) should be disposed of properly. Untreated refuse is unsightly and smelly and degrades both the quality of the environment and the quality of life in the community. It also provides a breeding ground for disease vectors, such as mosquitoes, flies and rats. If waste is not properly disposed of, animals can bring it close to the home and children can come into contact with disease vectors and pathogens. To be effective, solid waste disposal programmes require action at both household and community levels—if only a few households dispose of waste properly, the village environment may remain dirty and contaminated. Community members should decide how important solid waste management is and determine the best ways to achieve waste-management goals.

6.1 Strategies for solid waste management: minimizing waste and recycling

Key strategies for improving solid waste management and disposal are to minimize the waste generated by households, and to recycle waste whenever possible. To minimize waste, it is important that both the households and the community at large make a conscious decision to reduce the amount of waste they produce and actively participate in recycling. This may involve carrying food and other purchases in reusable bags, such as cloth bags, rather than using plastic bags. Minimizing waste may also entail sorting and recycling waste, which is discussed in more detail below and illustrated in Figure 6.1.

Solid wastes should be sorted for recycling, and for burying or burning. Recycling includes composting organic wastes, and reusing plastic and glass products as well as construction debris. It can offer both cost-saving and economic opportunities for communities. One way a community could generate additional revenue, for example, would be to sell paper waste to industries that use old paper in their manufacturing processes. Paper wastes can also be compacted into dense fuel briquettes and used for cooking to

Figure 6.1 **Separated wastes**

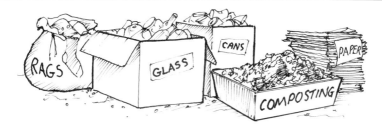

supplement firewood. This would also help reduce deforestation, which itself can adversely affect soil fertility and the quality of water sources. If used tyres are not recycled the best option may be to bury them, since burning produces toxic fumes. They should not be left as waste, because they can fill with rainwater and become breeding sites for insects that carry serious diseases.

6.2 Managing solid waste in households

Some low-cost methods for managing household solid waste are summarized below. More information may be available from local government staff, or from agencies such as NGOs and donor organizations.

6.2.1 Composting

Fruit and vegetable waste, animal dung and even leaves from trees can break down to form a valuable soil conditioner and fertilizer (compost). Household vegetable waste, for example, can be composted in a suitable container. After a few months the contents can be removed and used as fertilizer. An example of a household composting container is shown in Figure 6.2. A more sophisticated option is to use timber and chicken wire to construct a ventilated container that promotes composting. Again, vegetable waste is disposed of in the container until it is full, or until the compost is required.

6.2.2 Turning organic waste into fuel

Vegetable waste, including vegetable peelings and dried weeds, can be chopped up and compressed into small bricks and dried in the sun. Animal dung, too, can be spread thinly on the ground and dried in the sun. Once dried, the waste can be stored and used to replace charcoal or wood as a cooking fuel.

Figure 6.2 *Household composting container*

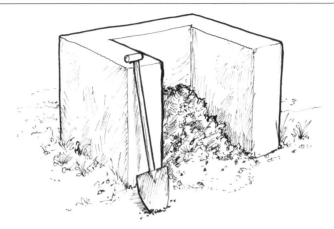

6.3 Managing solid waste in the community

Certain wastes are preferably managed at a community level. Some household items do not decompose and can cause injury if not properly disposed of. For example, neither glass nor plastics can be used in composting, and plastic gives off poisonous fumes when burned. Bones and metal items do decompose, but the process is very slow; batteries contain toxic chemicals. Bones, metal objects and broken glass can also be thrown into a latrine pit, but only if the pit is not going to be reused.

6.3.1 Communal refuse pit

A communal refuse pit is simply a pit dug near the community compound and filled with general refuse. The pit should not be located close to a water source, because toxic chemicals could leach into the water.

The disposal site itself should be fenced off to prevent access by scavenging animals. At the end of the day, new waste should be covered with a layer of clean soil 0.1 metre deep. When the pit is full, the waste should be covered with a final layer of soil to prevent flies from breeding.

6.3.2 Communal collection

Householders may transport their solid waste to the disposal site or communal collection may be organized. Communities themselves can organize waste collection, for example by purchasing a suitable vehicle and charging households for the service. If this is done, however, it is essential that the community members who perform the service are provided with protective equipment and are trained to handle waste safely. This type of approach provides employment and income to community households, improves the environment and reduces health risks.

Communal collection points are particularly important at places such as markets and bus stations, where large numbers of people congregate and food is prepared, sold and eaten. Communal containers, such as empty oil drums, skips or concrete bunkers, can be located strategically, so that solid waste is collected at a single site. If communal concrete bunkers are constructed, they should have holes at the base to encourage drainage away from the bunkers, but care must be taken not to cause contamination of either groundwater or surface water sources. Ideally, water from the waste bunkers should flow into the drainage system and be treated before it enters a river or stream.

It is preferable that vegetable waste is not disposed of in communal collection points unless these are emptied on a daily basis. Vegetable matter decomposes rapidly, is often very smelly and may cause significant contamination of groundwater sources.

All waste from communal collection points should be collected several times a week and taken to a designated disposal site. It can be transported in boxes, or by handcarts, animal carts, bicycles with box containers, tractors with trailers and skip-trucks. The waste should preferably be collected by staff wearing protective clothing and masks, who are trained in safe disposal methods.

6.4 **Managing special solid wastes**

Some solid wastes require special handling and their disposal should be carried out only by trained staff with proper clothing and equipment. Such wastes represent a special health risk and their proper disposal is essential for protecting health in the community. These wastes and their management are discussed in sections 6.4.1–6.4.3.

6.4.1 **Health care solid wastes**

Health care wastes can be generated both by medical facilities and by activities at home, such as changing bandages. Often, these wastes contain infectious pathogens; ideally they should be incinerated or safely buried immediately. Incineration can be carried out at a health centre or clinic, and it is preferable to use purpose-built incinerators with chimneys. However, simple home or community incinerators can be made from oil drums. If incineration is not an option, an alternative is to put bandages or other waste into a strong disinfectant. The person who does this must wear gloves. They should also wash their hands immediately after handling the waste, even though gloves were used. When bandages are to be reused, they should be thoroughly disinfected in strong bleach. If health care wastes are buried, they should be disposed of in a pit that restricts the access of people and animals. The pit should be built in the medical facility compound and should be surrounded by a fence; each layer of waste should be immediately covered with a layer of dirt. The pit should also be properly lined to prevent contamination of groundwater.

If needles must be used at home, for example because a person is a diabetic, they should be disinfected and disposed of properly. Used plastic syringes or their needles should never be reused, as this can cause serious illness. The needles should be blunted before disposal, to prevent them from becoming a hazard to others, and then burned or buried.

6.4.2 Slaughterhouse solid wastes

Slaughterhouse wastes contain decaying animal carcasses, blood and faecal matter, and they are a significant source of pathogens and bad odours. These wastes may also pollute water supplies. As slaughterhouse wastes represent a particular hazard, their collection and disposal should be carried out by trained staff and the wastes disposed of in properly maintained sites. If there are slaughterhouses in a community, community members should ensure that the local health authorities inspect the premises to ensure that proper procedures are followed.

6.4.3 Industrial solid wastes

Industrial wastes contain toxic chemicals that pose health risks and pollute the environment. While most industries will be located in towns, some small-scale industries, such as tanneries and mining operations, may be located in rural areas.

Tannery wastes, in particular, contain highly toxic metal compounds that cause both short- and long-term health problems. If water sources are polluted with tannery wastes, they may be unusable for many years, resulting in higher costs for drinking-water and adversely impacting health. If small-scale tanneries are located in a village, environmental protection agencies should be consulted about ways of reducing the risk of pollution.

Small-scale mining operations also use and produce toxic chemicals, such as mercury, and arsenic. These chemicals represent a serious health risk to the population, and if mining is carried out in a community, community members should seek advice on how to dispose of toxic chemicals properly. While it may not be possible for the community itself to set up disposal and treatment areas for industrial wastes, it is important that community members recognize the hazards of these wastes and request support to ensure that they are properly disposed of.

6.5 Chemical safety

Toxic chemicals are frequently used within a village and within homes. Pesticides, dips and inorganic fertilizers, for example, are used in agriculture, and toxic chemicals are commonly used in the repair of vehicles. In the home, chemicals are used as cleaning agents. Many of these chemicals are highly toxic and care should be taken to store, use and dispose of them safely. In particular, the manufacturers' instructions on use, storage and disposal should be carefully followed; these are usually marked on the packaging. If they are not, or if they are in a foreign language, advice on disposal should be sought from the suppliers, or the product should be avoided. If chemicals are past their "sell-by" date they should be avoided.

6.5.1 Storage of toxic chemicals

All chemicals should be kept in a safe place and out of the reach of children, for example by storing them in a locked cupboard. When chemicals are stored in houses, workshops or stores, individuals should be aware of the dangers posed by the chemicals, and poisonous chemicals should be clearly marked with a danger symbol recognizable by all community members. Chemical stores should remain locked when not in use and keys given only to individuals who must use the chemicals. Chemical stores should also be well ventilated, as many chemicals give off toxic fumes. With chlorine products, for example, there must be ventilation at the bottom of the building because chlorine is heavier than air and chlorine gas will accumulate at floor level. Local health and environment staff can be consulted about the safe storage and ventilation of chemicals.

For safety reasons, chemical stores should have a shower or washing system so that users can wash themselves immediately in the event of a toxic chemical spill. One option is to keep a full barrel of water close to the store for this purpose. When chemicals give off toxic fumes, breathing apparatus may also be required for people entering the store. Chemical stores should be located away from water sources to avoid the possibility of toxic chemicals infiltrating the soil and contaminating drinking-water supplies. Poorly stored agricultural chemicals in particular, such as fertilizers and pesticides, can get into the groundwater.

Figure 6.3 *Unhealthy use of agricultural chemicals*

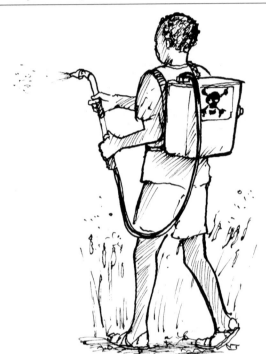

6.5.2 Handling toxic chemicals

All chemicals should be handled with great care. Most are toxic at some level and even though short-term exposure may not be particularly harmful, long-term exposure can cause serious health problems. For example, organophosphates in sheep dips can lead to heart and breathing problems, and to mental health problems. Consequently, agricultural workers should be trained in the use of chemicals. Training is usually carried out by agricultural extension workers and will normally include such topics as use of protective clothing, gloves and breathing apparatus. An example of bad practice in handling agricultural chemicals is shown in Figure 6.3. If there are any doubts regarding the safe handling and use of agricultural chemicals, workers should seek advice from local agricultural staff, otherwise the community may be exposed to serious health risks. If a toxic spill occurs, it should be contained as far as possible and the appropriate local or national environmental agency contacted.

6.5.3 **Chemicals in the home**

Many households use chemical cleaning products that can be harmful if not handled and stored correctly. Gloves and other protective wear should be worn when chemicals such as bleach are used, even if they are diluted. Fumes should not be inhaled, nor should the chemicals be allowed to enter the eyes or mouth, since many household chemicals are poisonous in sufficient amounts. Children are more likely to suffer accidents than adults, and chemicals should be stored in locked cupboards, out of reach of children as shown in Figure 6.4. If a chemical accident occurs in the home, medical advice should be sought immediately. With some chemicals, if detoxification is not carried out right away, death or permanent injury can result.

When insecticides are used in the home to control mosquitoes, flies and other insects, manufacturers' instructions must be followed and the products kept out of the reach of children. In a Healthy Village approach, however,

Figure 6.4 ***Keeping household chemicals secure**￼*

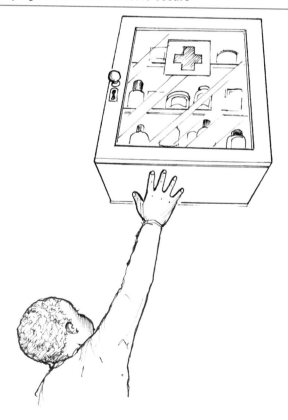

communities should be informed about alternative and more sustainable ways of insect control, such as draining insect breeding sites, screening houses, using impregnated mosquito nets and introducing fish that feed on mosquito larvae.

6.5.4 Disposal of toxic chemicals

Proper disposal of toxic chemicals requires responsibility and action at both household and community levels. In households where home chemicals are not safely disposed of, it is not simply the health of family members that is jeopardized; the health of all community members is placed at risk. Old chemicals should not be indiscriminately dumped in the environment, as this can pollute both soil and water, and the chemicals may give off toxic fumes. If it is suspected that toxic chemicals are being illegally dumped in a community, the local agency responsible for waste management or for the environment should be contacted immediately and community members should insist that preventive action be taken.

Chemicals should be disposed of according to manufacturers' guidance and if they have passed their "sell-by" date they should be collected by trained staff and disposed of at special sites. If there is any doubt about how to dispose of chemicals, local health and environment officials should be consulted.

CHAPTER 7

Housing quality

Good-quality housing is a key element for ensuring a healthy village. Poor housing can lead to many health problems, and is associated with infectious diseases (such as tuberculosis), stress and depression. Everyone should therefore have access to good-quality housing and a pleasant home environment that makes them happy and content. Specific aspects of housing quality are described in the following sections.

Problems associated with poor housing

- Cramped and crowded conditions give rise to poor hygiene by providing places for vermin to breed and transmit diseases via fleas, ticks and other vectors.

- Poor household hygiene leads to food and water contamination within the home.

- Poor indoor air quality leads to respiratory problems and inadequate lighting leads to eyesight problems.

- Stress is higher for individuals living in poor housing and poverty.

7.1 **Ventilation**

Adequate home ventilation is particularly important where wood, charcoal and dung are used for cooking or heating, since these fuels give off smoke that contains harmful chemicals and particulate matter. This can lead to respiratory problems, such as bronchitis and asthma, and make tuberculosis transmission easier. Women and small children are particularly at risk from poor ventilation if they spend long periods within the home or in cooking areas. Where cooking is done indoors, it is essential that smoke and fumes be removed from the house quickly and efficiently. Ventilation may be improved by constructing houses with a sufficient number of windows, particularly in cooking areas. Alternatively, houses can be constructed using bricks with holes drilled through them ("air-bricks"), which allow fresh air to circulate within the house.

Figure 7.1 *House with good ventilation and light*

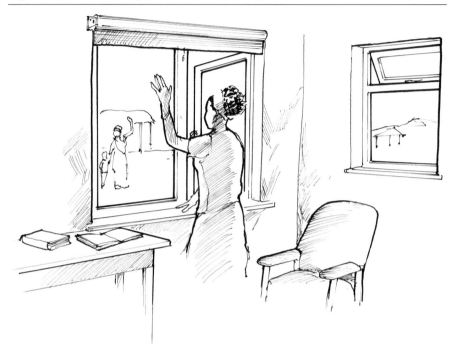

7.2 Lighting

Poor indoor lighting can have many harmful effects on health and well-being. A poorly lit working environment in the home can lead to eyesight problems, for example. This is a particular concern for women working in indoor cooking areas. Poor lighting within the home can also make people feel more depressed. These problems can be remedied by adding windows to the house to increase the amount of natural light, which is much stronger than light from candles or lamps, as shown in Figure 7.1. In communities where it is important that privacy within the home is maintained, windows can be located where it is difficult for people to see into the house, or constructed with a mesh or lattice work which allows light to enter while guarding privacy. Increasing natural light is also important for home cleanliness: if a house is dark, it is more difficult to see dust and dirt and thus more difficult to clean properly.

7.3 Disease vectors in the home

Unless homes are kept clean and steps taken to prevent insects from entering, the homes can become infested with disease vectors. In eastern

Figure 7.2 **Example of a house with unhygienic practices**

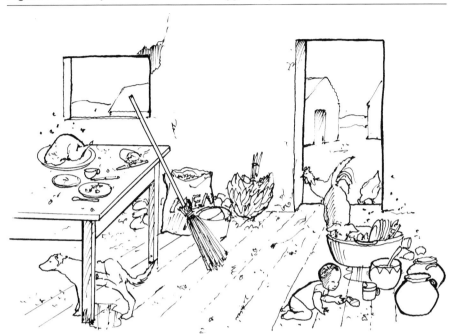

Mediterranean areas, for example, sandflies thrive in the dirt inside houses and transmit leishmaniasis; and in Central and South America, triatomid bugs live in the cracks of walls and in thatched roofs and transmit American trypanosomiasis (Chagas disease). Insect disease vectors can be reduced by keeping food covered and properly disposing of waste. If mosquitoes or flies are a problem, windows and doors should be covered with mesh screens and kept shut at night, and mosquito nets placed over beds. Cleanliness within and around home areas significantly reduces the risk of disease transmission. Examples of bad and good household hygiene are shown in Figures 7.2 and 7.3.

7.4 **Overcrowding in homes**

Overcrowding in homes causes ill-health because it makes disease transmission easier and because the lack of private space causes stress. Overcrowding is related to socioeconomic level, and the poor often have little choice but to live in cramped conditions. In principle, increasing the number of rooms in a house should improve the health of the people who live there, but increasing house size is often difficult. Careful planning of family size can also help to reduce overcrowding. If community members feel that overcrowding is a

Figure 7.3 **Example of a house with hygienic practices**

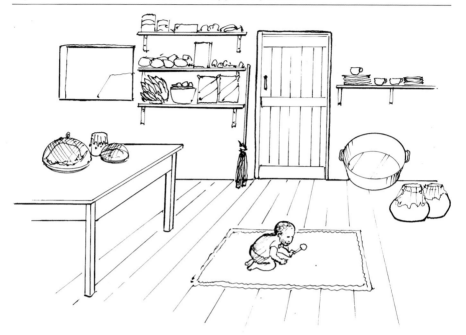

problem, they can take the initiative and press landlords to provide more space for tenants at affordable prices. This may necessitate working with local government and pressure groups to ensure that the housing laws and tenancy agreements are revised, and that everyone has access to houses adequate for their family size.

CHAPTER 8

Personal, domestic and community hygiene

Good hygiene is an important barrier to many infectious diseases, including the faecal–oral diseases, and it promotes better health and well-being. To achieve the greatest health benefits, improvements in hygiene should be made concurrently with improvements in the water supply and sanitation, and be integrated with other interventions, such as improving nutrition and increasing incomes. The next sections discuss how to improve personal and community hygiene practices that help to prevent the spread of faecal–oral diseases.

If wastewater is not disposed of effectively it can serve as a breeding ground for mosquitoes. People may also slip and fall in muddy puddles, and children may play in them and risk waterborne illness.

8.1 Personal and domestic hygiene

8.1.1 Handwashing

Proper handwashing is one of the most effective ways of preventing the spread of diarrhoeal diseases. Pathogens cannot be seen on hands, and water alone is not always sufficient to remove them. Soap and wood ash are both cleansing and disinfecting agents when used with water and can be used to kill pathogens on hands and utensils. The most important times that hands should be washed with soap and water are:

- After defecating.
- After cleaning a child who has defecated.
- Before eating or handling food.

Promoting good personal hygiene often requires that community members are mobilized towards this goal and awareness is raised about how to achieve it. It is important that hygiene education programmes do more than simply tell people that if they do not wash their hands they will become sick because of pathogens they cannot see. This rarely works. Instead, education programmes should try different methods to maximize community participation in the programmes and to encourage people to promote good hygiene. Some methods for promoting hygiene and health are discussed in the next chapter.

To encourage handwashing to become part of the daily routine, suitable facilities must be located near to places such as latrines and kitchens, where they will be needed. If running water is available, the facilities should include a tap and a sink as well as soap. Hands may also be washed at a tap stand as shown in Figures 8.1 and 8.2. If running water is not available, an oil can or bucket fitted with a tap is a simple way of providing handwashing facilities; the larger the container, the less frequently it will need filling. Some containers are mounted on stands with a ledge for soap. A leaking container (such as a tin can with holes in its base) can also be used to scoop water from the water storage container and provide a stream of running water for handwashing. Another approach involves a suspended container that, when tipped, pours water onto the hands of the user. The system can easily be made from plastic cooking oil containers. Soap itself can be kept clean by suspending it above the ground on a string.

8.1.2 Bathing

Regular bathing and laundering are important for cleanliness and good personal appearance. They also prevent hygiene-related diseases such as scabies, ringworm, trachoma, conjunctivitis and louse-borne typhus. Educational and promotional activities can encourage bathing and laundering, but increasing the number of washing facilities and locating them conveniently may be more effective. Bathing with soap is an important means of preventing the transmission of trachoma—an illness that can cause blindness and other eyesight problems. Children's faces in particular should be washed regularly and thoroughly. If a child has trachoma, a special towel or tissue should be used to wipe or dry the child's face; the towel should never be used for other children because of the risk of transmitting the disease. Ideally, programmes that promote bathing should be combined with a programme to reduce the numbers of flies, which spread trachoma and other diseases, and to improve sanitation.

For people to bathe thoroughly they must use sufficient water, but it may be difficult to promote the use of more water for washing if water supplies are distant and water must be collected by hand. Moreover, many traditional bathing practices do not use water efficiently and ensuring cleanliness may be difficult. By modifying existing practices, such as by encouraging the use of water containers with taps, it may be possible to improve the efficiency of water use. Community shower units, with separate facilities for men and women, can also become income-generating enterprises in larger villages, but the facilities require careful maintenance and must be conveniently located. Operators should also allay concerns about voyeurism, which may be

Figure 8.1 *Handwashing using a tap*

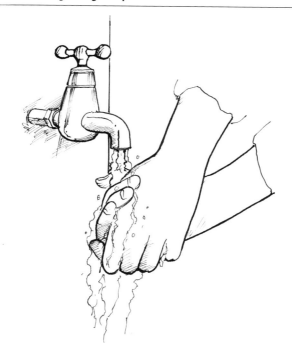

Figure 8.2 *Handwashing at a standpost*

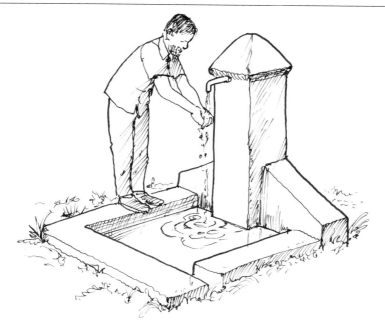

particularly important to women. Such problems are best resolved through discussion within the community.

8.1.3 Laundering

To promote laundering of clothes and bedding, laundry slabs or sinks can be constructed near water points. They should be large enough to wash bedding and other bulky items and be situated so that water drains away from the laundry area and away from the water source. Locating laundry places in natural water bodies, streams and irrigation canals is best avoided if possible, since this practice can contribute to the transmission of schistosomiasis.

8.2 Community hygiene

Some health measures can be undertaken only by the community as a whole; these include water source protection, proper disposal of solid waste and excreta, wastewater drainage, controlling animal rearing and market hygiene. Some of these issues have been described in earlier sections. Individual community members play an important role in community hygiene, and have a responsibility to their neighbours and to the community to promote good health and a clean environment. For example, everyone in the village must keep their houses and compounds clean, because one dirty house can affect many conscientious neighbours and contribute to the spread of disease. Community leaders can promote cleanliness in the home by regularly checking on village households and by using by-laws to encourage household maintenance.

8.2.1 Markets

Markets often represent a health hazard because foodstuffs may not be stored properly and because the markets may lack basic services, such as water supply, sanitation, solid waste disposal and drainage. Ideally, markets should have several taps to provide traders and customers with ready access to safe water for drinking and washing. Many vegetable and fruit sellers regularly sprinkle their produce with water, and it is important that they have access to clean water for this. The sanitation facilities should also be appropriate for the number of people who will visit the market, with separate facilities for men and women. Water and sanitation facilities for a market are often relatively easy to support by charging a small user fee, or by using part of the market fee to pay for such services. If people are charged a fee to use the facilities, discounts can be offered to traders who already support the facilities through their market fee.

Foodstuffs sold at the market should be inspected daily by health officials. This is particularly important for meat and fish, which should be inspected before sale to ensure that they have been prepared according to national regulations and that they do not contain pathogens or other contaminants. Markets usually generate a lot of solid waste and it is important that it is disposed of properly, to prevent vermin such as rats and insects from feeding and breeding among it. The layout of market stalls should thus allow easy access for vehicles that collect waste and clean the area. Solid waste should be collected and disposed of daily, and preferably more often. Strategically located waste bins (often concrete bunkers) can make this more effective. Market areas should also be properly drained to prevent flooding and insect breeding.

Successful refuse collection in west Africa

In one west African market, refuse collection was effective because there were enough disposal points, and because the market was closed for a short time each day to allow waste to be collected and the market to be cleaned. This made the market safer and more attractive to customers.

Markets function most effectively when they have legal status, with market fees and supervision, preferably by health officials based at the market. Well-run markets tend to have strong traders' associations and good links between market associations and local service providers. Market traders can have a strong voice in improving conditions, since they generate significant income for communities and provide essential food distribution services. Traders' associations can set up standards for the market, can successfully manage water and sanitation facilities, and can organize regular waste collection. If markets are held regularly, community members should seek advice and support from local health staff on issues such as setting up an association, establishing trading standards and penalties for contravention, and on lobbying for service provision. As markets grow, the management of services often gets easier because the growing number of fees collected provides more income for services.

8.2.2 Animal rearing

In many communities animal rearing is a means of generating food high in protein content and nutritional value, and for generating additional income. Animals can also provide many other products, such as leather and fuel, that improve the quality of life. However, if it is not practised safely, animal rearing can have negative effects on the health of the community. Animals should always be kept away from households, particularly cooking areas and drinking-water sources, since their excreta contain pathogens that can contaminate food and water. Preferably, animals should be kept in compounds at least 100 metres from water sources and 10 metres from houses. Animal waste should be disposed of properly, away from homes and water sources, or be used as a fertilizer. It is also best that animals are slaughtered away from households and water sources, since the offal and wastes may introduce contamination. Slaughtering must be carried out by qualified individuals who follow the country laws governing slaughter practices..

Some disease vectors prefer animal hosts to humans. Pigs, for example, can be reservoirs of Japanese encephalitis, dogs can be reservoirs of leishmaniasis, and some mosquitoes prefer to feed on cattle rather than humans. Placing animal shelters between mosquito breeding places and the village may therefore provide some protection against malaria transmission.

8.3 Food hygiene

Contaminated food represents one of the greatest health risks to a population and is a leading cause of disease outbreaks and transmission. Food that is kept too long can go bad and contain toxic chemicals or pathogens, and foodstuffs that are eaten raw, such as fruits or vegetables, can become contaminated by dirty hands, unclean water or flies. Improperly prepared food can also cause chemical poisoning: cassava leaf that has not been properly pounded and cooked, for example, may contain dangerous levels of cyanide. To promote good health, therefore, food should be properly stored and prepared. Ways in which communities can prevent health risks from food are discussed in the following sections.

8.3.1 Food preparation in the home

As most food is likely to be prepared in the home, it is important that families understand the principles of basic hygiene and know how to prepare food safely. Before preparing food, hands should be washed with soap or ash. Raw fruit and vegetables should not be eaten unless they are first peeled or washed with clean water. It is also important to cook food properly, particularly meat. Both cattle and pigs host tapeworms that can be transferred to humans through improperly cooked meat; for this reason, raw meat should never be eaten. Eggs, too, must be cooked properly before eating, since they may contain salmonella, a virulent pathogen. The kitchen itself should be kept clean and waste food disposed of carefully to avoid attracting vermin, such as rats and mice, that may transmit disease. Keeping food preparation surfaces clean is critical, because harmful organisms can grow on these surfaces and contaminate food.

Fresh meat should be cooked and eaten on the same day, unless it can be stored in a refrigerator; if not, it should be thrown away. Cooked food should be eaten while it is still hot and should not be left to stand at room temperature for long periods of time, since this provides a good environment for pathogens to grow. Food that is ready to eat should be covered as shown in Figure 8.3 to keep off flies and should be thrown away if not eaten within 12–16 hours. If food must be stored after cooking, it should be kept covered and in a cool place, such as a refrigerator. If a refrigerator is not available, food can be stored on ice blocks or in a preservative such as pickling vinegar or salt. Food that is already prepared, or food that is to be eaten raw, must not come into contact with raw meat as this may contain pathogens that can contaminate the other foods (particularly if slaughtering was not carried out hygienically).

8.3.2 Eating-houses

In many rural communities food is bought and consumed at eating-houses (cafes, restaurants or cantinas). If basic health and safety rules for storing, preparing and handling food are not followed in the eating-houses, these places will represent a health hazard for the customers and may cause serious disease outbreaks. The most important aspects of food hygiene in these establishments relate to sanitation, water supply and personal cleanliness:

Figure 8.3 **Storing food properly**

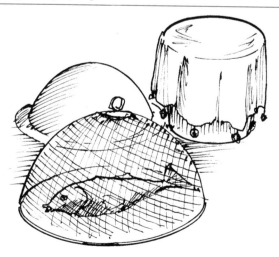

- Eating-houses should have clean water for washing and drinking, and separate sanitation facilities, away from the kitchen area, for customers, cooks and food-handlers.
- The staff should have clean uniforms each day and have regular medical check-ups.
- Food should be freshly prepared daily and any that is spilled or not used should be disposed of.
- The kitchens and eating areas must be kept clean and free of vermin and insects.
- Eating-houses should also be well-ventilated, with adequate lighting, and have procedures for dealing with fires and accidents. For example, the eating area should not be too crowded, to allow customers easy exit in the event of a fire.

Most countries have legislation covering eating-houses and their operation. As a rule, eating-houses require official approval before they can operate and are subject to regular checks. These checks are likely to be increased in times of epidemics. The community should recognize that eating-houses must be properly run and maintained to ensure that they do not become a source of disease. Eating-houses should be periodically checked, for example by health officials, to make sure that the establishments do not pose health risks. If a community member suspects an eating-house of posing a health hazard, he/she should request an inspection by the appropriate local health authorities.

8.3.3 Street food-vendors

Street food-vendors are common in urban and periurban areas, but they also operate in rural areas, particularly if there is a market or community fair with bars and other drinking establishments. Although people enjoy food from these vendors, in many cases the food is of poor quality and it represents a serious health risk. A study in one African city, for example, found that 98% of the street vendors had faecal contamination on their hands and food, a situation that is likely to be the same for food vendors in other cities and villages. In part, this is because the street vendors have little or no access to safe water supplies or sanitation facilities, and they commonly cook and handle food with dirty hands. Raw foodstuffs, too, cannot be kept in safe storage places and are easily contaminated by vermin and insects. Moreover, the street vendors often keep cooked food at ambient (environmental) temperatures for prolonged periods of time and may heat the food only slightly before serving. All these factors may make the food from street vendors dangerous.

Where street food-vendors are legal, they should be regulated by the health authorities. Often they are not legal, however, and in these cases steps should be taken to promote their safe management of food and, where necessary, to prevent them from selling their food. This may be difficult if the demand for street food is high, and it may be necessary to work closely with local health authorities. Street vendors should be encouraged to locate close to water points and sanitation facilities where they can keep hands and food clean. Community members can also work with vendors to ensure that food is prepared and eaten immediately, rather than being kept unrefrigerated for long periods.

8.3.4 Promoting nutrition

A healthy and well-balanced diet is essential for good health. When there is not enough food, or if the diet does not contain the right balance of foodstuffs, people become more prone to illness and may become undernourished or malnourished. Children, in particular, are vulnerable to poor nutrition. Undernourishment and malnourishment can lower their resistance and make them more likely to suffer from infectious diseases. Often, children will eat only small amounts of food if it is spicy, even if it is nutritious, and it is important to make children's food less spicy than adult food. Also, because their stomachs are small, children can eat only small portions and need to be fed more frequently than healthy adults. It is also important that children are fed not just foods high in starch or carbohydrate (for instance rice or cassava). Although these foods can quickly make a child feel full, he or she may become malnourished if other key foodstuffs are not eaten. A well-balanced diet usually has a mixture of food with protein (for example beans, peas, meat, fish or eggs), carbohydrates (such as maize, potatoes, cassava, rice and many other staple foods), vitamins (such as vegetables, fish, fruits or milk), and some fats or oils (such as cooking oil). Sometimes not all these foods are available and it is important that community members ask health workers how to make best use of available foods for a balanced diet.

In many situations, nutrition can be improved by changing agricultural or gardening practices. Often, even small plots of land can provide nutritious food provided that the right crops are grown. Health workers or agricultural extension workers can be asked for advice about which crops to grow to provide community members with well-balanced diets. It is not possible here to give a full discussion of the nutritional value of foods, or of what constitutes a well-balanced diet. This is an enormous subject and is covered in more detail in materials developed by other programmes and organizations. However, it is important that communities request advice and support for improving nutrition. Many organizations that provide advice and support to nutrition programmes are listed in Annex 1.

CHAPTER 9

Promoting hygiene

The goal of hygiene promotion is to help people to understand and develop good hygiene practices, so as to prevent disease and promote positive attitudes towards cleanliness. Several community development activities can be used to achieve this goal, including education and learning programmes, encouraging community management of environmental health facilities, and social mobilization and organization. Hygiene promotion is not simply a matter of providing information. It is more a dialogue with communities about hygiene and related health problems, to encourage improved hygiene practices. Some key steps for establishing a hygiene promotion project, possibly with support from an outside agency, are listed in the text box below.

Establishing a hygiene promotion project

- Evaluate whether current hygiene practices are good/safe.
- Plan which good hygiene practices to promote.
- Implement a health promotion programme that meets community needs and is understandable by everyone.
- Monitor and evaluate the programme to see whether it is meeting targets.

9.1 Assessing hygiene practices

To assess whether good hygiene is practised by your community, some of the methods discussed in section 2.2 can be used. It is particularly important to identify behaviours that spread pathogens. The following are the riskiest behaviours:

- The unsafe disposal of faeces.
- Not washing hands with soap after defecating.
- The unsafe collection and storage of water.

Key questions for assessing hygiene

- What "risky" practices are widespread in the community?
- How many people employ risky practices and who are they?
- Which risky practices can be altered?
- What motivates those who currently use "safe" practices?
- Who influences them?
- What communication channels are available?
- Which communication channels are trusted for hygiene messages?

9.2 Planning hygiene promotion projects

The entire community should be involved in a hygiene promotion project, but this is likely to mean that different groups within the community will have different perceptions and priorities. Women's priorities are particularly important, since women usually ensure that good hygiene is practised in the home. It is crucial to take these different priorities into account and make realistic plans. By consulting all community members, it is possible to identify priorities and achieve solutions more relevant to the whole community.

When identifying community members to carry out hygiene education, it is important to consider the amount of time they will spend on promotional activities and how they will be compensated. The duties and skills required by prospective promoters should also be clearly identified. Existing health staff and teachers may be appropriate as hygiene education providers, but they may not have the time to commit to additional activities or have the skills to carry out activities on sensitive subjects. Other community members may perform hygiene education activities well, but may require training. In such cases, local government bodies and other agencies should be contacted to provide the necessary training and support. Usually, the most effective skills in a promoter are an ability to communicate well with the target group and an understanding of constraints that cause people not to adopt safe practices. People who cannot read or write should not be excluded as promoters if these skills are not required, since that may exclude older women who are respected in the community and have plenty of life experience.

There is no hard-and-fast rule for the ratio of hygiene promoters to community members, but it is generally considered that one community promoter can adequately cover about 1000 community members, provided that it is easy to move between households. Community promoters can be supervised by an outside agency or by local government officials, but the community itself should also be involved to ensure that the programme is effective and responsive to local needs.

9.3 Implementing hygiene promotion projects

Flexibility is essential when implementing a hygiene promotion project. Different community members may need different information and support, and the project as a whole may need to change as it develops.

9.3.1 Building community capacity

To promote hygiene within a community it is not enough simply to provide messages about hygiene; the capacity of the community to analyse situations and initiate changes must also be improved. In this sense, hygiene promotion is comparable to community development activities. Building community capacity may involve:

- Operating and maintaining water and sanitation facilities.
- Organizing and supporting community groups and committees.
- Helping communities to analyse their current hygiene and sanitation.
- Negotiating agreements and settlements between development partners.
- Encouraging the private sector to develop water, sanitation and hygiene products.

9.3.2 Organizing groups and committees

Groups and committees, such as water and sanitation user groups, may be required to perform hygiene-related tasks, and it may be difficult to involve all members of the community in these groups. Women, for example, may not be able to serve on water and sanitation committees, yet fulfilling their needs is of paramount importance to the work of the committees. In some cases, hygiene promotion staff may be able to encourage the representation of women on committees, but it may be more appropriate to have separate committees for women. When these are established, however, there must be a link to the overall community committee responsible for managing the water and sanitation facilities, so that women's opinions influence management. The women may require special training to develop their confidence and communication skills and to effectively represent women's interests on committees.

9.3.3 **Situation analysis**

Before a project with a community is started, information about the current hygiene situation should be collected and analysed. This will help to guide project activities and provide a baseline against which changes can be measured. The information collected from a project will also form the basis of other hygiene promotion activities. Situation analysis should not be undertaken by hygiene promotion staff alone, but should involve the entire community, both during the project and afterwards. Hygiene promotion staff can share findings with the community, and help community members to analyse information and identify solutions to problems.

9.3.4 **Communication and education**

Communication and education activities include selecting appropriate hygiene messages; identifying the target groups for those messages; identifying effective communication methods; preparing communication materials; and communicating the messages. Selecting the appropriate hygiene messages and identifying target audiences require an analysis of information collected from the community. Mothers are often designated as the primary target audience, since they are usually the main caregivers for young children and are most influential in a family setting. While targeting mothers may be useful for influencing change at household level, there is also a need to involve the immediate family and other people who influence women's behaviour.

Accessing target audiences

- Who are the members of each target group?
- Where are they?
- How many of them are there?
- What languages do they speak?
- Who listens to the radio or watches television regularly?
- What proportion can read?
- Do they read newspapers?
- To which organizations and groups do they belong?
- Which channels of communication do they like and trust?

Figure 9.1 *Health education group*

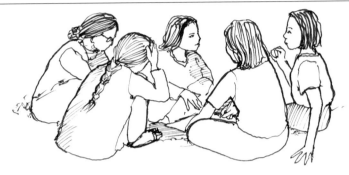

Hygiene education messages can be communicated in different ways, including posters, drama and storytelling, mass media messages, group discussions (Figure 9.1) and home visits. Some methods, such as the use of mass media and posters, communicate messages to large numbers of people. Other approaches emphasize the need to work with small groups, through meetings and household visits. No single method is always effective, however. Most health education works best when interventions are made at different levels and use a mixture of awareness-raising tools, and when they focus on individual activities, such as "child-to-child" programmes or home visits by health educators. Getting households and community members involved in learning about hygiene is often crucial for improving hygiene practices and reducing the risks to health. The messages should be understandable by the target audience. This can be accomplished by first testing educational materials on small pilot groups. More information on hygiene communication and education can be obtained from the agencies and materials listed in Annexes 1 and 2.

9.4 **Monitoring and evaluating hygiene projects**

Regular review of hygiene education projects by community members ensures that issues important to the community are covered. Reviews can evaluate whether community members are uncertain or confused about hygiene messages and whether they need further hygiene information. The results of reviews also provide feedback to hygiene educators for improving the programmes. Community members should decide on the frequency with which hygiene education activities are evaluated. Meetings could be held every 1–2 weeks, with assessment based on agreed goals set at each meeting, or less frequently (every 3–6 months) with more lengthy discussions at each meeting. When outside donors have provided funds, they may have their own requirements for monitoring and evaluating the information collected, so it is important that the community members are clear about how such evaluations will be performed and what role the community will play.

Evaluation activities

- Try to decide what information is needed. This may require reaching a consensus with all concerned individuals and organizations, a process that may involve lengthy negotiations.

- Identify who will carry out the investigations. This, too, can be a lengthy process and depends on the availability and willingness of individuals to help.

- Select tools for collecting information. (Who has the information, what form is it in and who will collect it?)

- Organize logistic arrangements. Try to make sure that everyone involved in the project is contacted and provided with necessary information in a timely manner. The staff or community members undertaking the evaluation may need guidance on how they should collect information and how they should respond to evaluation issues.

- Review findings with investigators. This may need to be coordinated by a committee of representatives from different stakeholder groups.

- Provide feedback to all stakeholders about investigators' findings. Different reports will probably be needed for different stakeholders.

9.4.1 Deciding what information is needed

Developing a framework of questions is the first step in monitoring and evaluating a hygiene education programme, and the framework should include a measurement of what has happened and how it has happened. Some of the most common questions to consider are:

- **Appropriateness.** Are project activities the right ones? Do they provide solutions to the most important problems?
- **Effectiveness.** How well are the different activities carried out?
- **Costs.** What does the project cost? What contributions come from the community and are they acceptable?
- **Participation.** Who attends project activity meetings? Are all groups represented in planning, implementing and evaluating the activities?
- **Sustainability**. Can activities be sustained on a continuing basis? If external agencies provide funds, can the community sustain activities after funding has ceased?
- **Unintended outcomes.** Are there outcomes (positive or negative) that were not intended?

9.4.2 **Selecting project investigators**

The community should be actively involved in any assessment, including the collection and review of information, and should identify individuals within the community to carry out the assessment. Individuals from external support agencies may also assist in the evaluation, which could bring new perspectives to the project and facilitate the collection and review of information. Selecting community members to undertake the assessment requires careful planning; to ensure that assessment results are reliable it is usually best to involve a mix of community members. This mix can include community members involved in the health education project, as well as those who are not actively involved but who have a good understanding of project goals.

9.4.3 **Selecting tools for collecting information**

The type of monitoring and evaluation tools chosen will depend on the type of information to be collected. This section describes some of the tools available.

Assessment tools

Assessment tools can be used at various points during the project to determine whether interventions are improving community hygiene. Focus group discussions, for example, can be useful for revealing community views and for solving problems that arise during discussions. For more quantitative assessments, questionnaires can be used to record activities and behaviours. The assessment tools should be carefully selected so that the collected information is appropriate to the purposes of the evaluation.

Self-monitoring forms

By using self-monitoring forms, households can monitor their own hygiene practices, or can monitor the incidence of an illness over time. The forms can then be collected and discussed with householders, either individually or as part of a group discussion. Health educators can also monitor their own activities using self-monitoring forms and they should meet regularly to discuss problems and successes. Self-monitoring forms should be easily understandable by users and by individuals who collect and analyse the information.

Trainers' assessment forms

Training sessions should be regularly assessed to maintain their quality. Again, the trainers' assessment forms should be easily understandable by everyone who collects and analyses the information. One way of assessing participants' attitudes towards a training course is to ask them to write down on a flip-chart one positive thing and one negative thing about the course. For those unable to write, a series of pictures representing feelings could be provided and the participants asked to mark those that best represent their own feelings about the training course.

9.4.4 Reviewing project findings

A review committee can be set up to manage the progress of the project and to discuss the implications of its findings; a hygiene committee, for example, could act as the reviewers. From the outset, committee members should be aware of the amount of time that the committee work will entail and understand the purpose of the evaluations. If the evaluation is important mainly to a donor or funding organization, the information collected may need to be representative of the community as a whole and its relevance for improving community hygiene clearly stated against the project goals. However, it may also be important for the evaluation to be used as a means of discussing the direction of the programme and of identifying how the effectiveness could be improved. If the evaluation is geared more towards the community, it can be used to generate further debate about the importance of the hygiene promotion programme and how it can be enhanced by the community itself.

9.4.5 Feedback and dissemination of findings

Information gathered during monitoring and evaluation activities should be shared with the wider community and other interested parties. This is best accomplished by holding group discussions with different sections of the community. Feedback can also be accomplished by posting notices at meeting places, or by presenting the information in the form of a drama. Written information should be summarized in no more than a couple of pages and illustrated with graphs, figures, pictograms and pictures. If information is shared with the community and other concerned people, discussions about progress can lead to new project targets or even to different types of projects.

CHAPTER 10

Providing health care

In any community, people become ill and require access to health care facilities and treatment. The problem may be physical, such as diarrhoea, fever or injury, or mental, e.g. psychosis, epilepsy or a learning difficulty. Women have special needs related to pregnancy and childbirth, and children require immunization against common diseases. Regardless of the nature of the health issue, the health outcomes depend to a large degree on individuals' ability to access health care services. Unfortunately, health services are often planned without consulting the community members who use and pay for such services, particularly in rural areas. To counter this, and to meet community demands for accessible, affordable services, community members should be actively involved in their planning. Health centres should attract the community (see Figure 10.1).

The way in which people deal with illness is also an important factor in health care. Most people initially treat ill-health within the home and seek outside help only when the problem continues or becomes severe. Such help may not necessarily come from qualified medical personnel; it can also come from local pharmacists or medicine sellers, traditional healers, religious leaders and friends. Often, seeking medical advice from qualified personnel is the last resort. This can happen for many reasons, such as that an individual does not consider the problem to be severe or "medical" in nature, or that the value of medical advice is not appreciated. Sometimes, there is simply mistrust of the medical profession.

Consequently, when planning health care interventions, it is important first to understand current health practices, as well as community needs: which health care services are available, what type of service the community wants and where health facilities should be located. This can be achieved through community discussions using participatory learning techniques with different community groups—defined by age, gender, wealth and ethnic/religious affiliation. The purpose is to generate a reliable picture of community needs and ensure that the services provided will be equitable, accessible and affordable.

Figure 10.1 *Rural health centre*

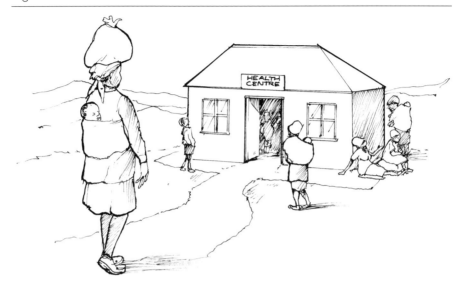

Providing health care services

- Health care facilities (rural clinics, health centres) should be within easy walking distance of the community, particularly for women and children.

- Outreach or primary health care workers, such as health visitors and promoters, can be valuable front-line community health workers if they are provided with adequate training and support, particularly if they come from the community itself.

- Other health service providers (pharmacists, medicine sellers, traditional healers) can provide additional health advice and care if they are given adequate training and support, and are supervised by medical staff.

- Referral systems between different levels of health care (primary, secondary and tertiary) should be clear and comprehensible to both users and providers. The reasons for referrals are often unclear to the users, which can provoke anxiety and lead to non-attendance. In addition, many primary- and secondary-level health care workers may not understand how to refer a patient to higher levels of service, or may not recognize symptoms of more severe illness, which leads to dangerous delays in referral.

10.1 Establishing community health care programmes

When community health care services are established, it is essential that the primary health care be effective and efficient. Community members can lobby local service providers to put primary health care workers in the community, as well as identify community members who could be trained to provide health advice. Other people who can provide health advice to the community, such as pharmacists or medicine sellers, birth attendants and traditional healers, should also be identified. Local service providers can be lobbied to provide additional training and support for these people if necessary. To be effective, health care workers should be acceptable to different community groups and have unrestricted access to the population. Women, for example, may not consider male health care workers to be acceptable for certain issues, and vice versa. Primary health care workers should also have sufficient knowledge and support to recognize illnesses that are beyond their ability to treat, and be able to refer patients to higher-level health care facilities for expert advice and treatment.

The role of pharmacists and medicine sellers in malaria treatment

In south Asia, WHO has promoted the use of local pharmacists and medicine sellers to provide treatment for malaria. They have been trained to recognize malaria symptoms, to prescribe the correct drug dosages, and to advise patients on whether they should seek expert advice. The programme has proved popular with communities, and with the medicine sellers and pharmacists, and it has reduced the burden on over-stretched health services.

The following questionnaire can help community members to determine whether current health services are adequate. If the community lacks adequate access to health services, a strategy for improving the services should be developed and presented to local service providers. Presenting a concrete plan for improving health services, rather than simply complaining that they are inadequate, will enable service providers to plan the necessary services better.

Are current health services adequate?

- Where is the nearest health centre to the community? Can women and children walk to it within one hour?
- Do trained health workers visit the community? What treatment and health advice can they offer?

- Do health workers provide health education by visiting households and schools, or by attending community meetings?

- Is there a pharmacist or medicine seller in the community or in a nearby community? What medicines can be obtained and what advice is provided? Do the pharmacists or medicine sellers receive supervision or support? Do community members consider them to be helpful in treating disease?

- If community members become sick, do they have access to drugs and other treatments?

- What sort of health service provision would the community like to have?

10.2 Factors that influence the type of health care that people seek

When people are sick many cultural and societal factors influence whether and where they seek health care and from whom. For example, it may be difficult for women to approach male health workers for certain problems. On the other hand, individuals in the community who are perceived as wise, or likely to have the required information, may be trusted by most community members. Too often, traditional ways of treating health problems are discounted by people outside a community who try to impose "western" or orthodox models of health care, with their emphasis on medication. However, if the illness is ascribed to angry gods or bad spirits, for example, this approach may not be perceived as effective and community members will be unlikely to seek orthodox health care; indigenous healers or religious leaders may be consulted instead.

The societal context of a disease, too, can affect whether people seek medical advice. In communities where communicable diseases are common, diarrhoea may not be viewed as a major problem unless it is severe. Frequent mild cases of malaria may not lead the sufferer to seek medical assistance, even though malaria can be a life-threatening disease. As a result, people often do not seek treatment and continue to have poor health.

For many reasons, therefore, it is important to work with a community to find out where individuals go for health advice and why. By understanding what help can be provided by different health care workers and how different people can work together, the best possible health care can be provided. This can be accomplished either by formal discussions or in more informal settings. By working with community members it will be possible to set up a referral system that includes all community health providers and to ensure that all providers have standard codes of practice.

Who provides community health advice?

- Are there any traditional healers or birth attendants in the community?
- What sort of advice do they provide?
- Do any problems arise from using traditional healers?
- Are there any health workers in the community?
- What services do they offer?
- Where do men mostly go to seek advice about their health or treatment?
- Where do women usually go to seek advice about their health or treatment?
- Where do families usually take their children when they are sick?
- Are boys taken to different people from girls?

10.3 Encouraging and sustaining the use of health services

For the cultural and societal reasons discussed in section 10.2, it can be difficult to change the way people seek health advice. To accomplish change, health care services must be easily available, since people are less likely to use good health services if they are distant from the community. If the community has been actively involved in planning and selecting the health services, it is also more likely that community members will use them. All community members should therefore be involved in the planning process, not simply community leaders. Community leaders may desire a certain level of health service, but if the rest of the community feels the service does not meet their needs, the result may be expensive services that are not used.

To sustain the use of health services, continuing campaigns in the community and in schools may be required. Educational messages through posters and the mass media can be part of larger campaigns within the community. Regular community meetings can also be held between outreach workers, influential people within the community, and community groups or households. A key strategy is to allow people to express their concerns about the health services. It may be, for example, that families do not use the available service because service providers have been rude or aggressive, or because the facility is not open at convenient times. Service providers and communities should therefore maintain a dialogue and find compromises that meet community demands but also reflect the capacity of the service.

10.4 Immunization of children

Vaccines are available for some major infectious childhood diseases, including measles, poliomyelitis, tuberculosis, diphtheria, tetanus, whooping cough (pertussis), mumps and rubella (German measles). However, all children in a community should have the full course of immunization for these diseases. If a child contracts a disease it is not just his or her health that is at risk: there is a risk of an outbreak within the community, and these diseases can be fatal or cause complications such as blindness, infertility, partial paralysis and stunting.

For the majority of the childhood diseases, it is most effective to immunize children at a young age (preferably under 1 year), usually by means of a series of injections or oral vaccines as shown in Figure 10.2. Most countries make immunization programmes available to communities at no cost through local health centres, although some may offer immunization services only on certain days. In other cases, mobile teams visit communities on certain days to carry out immunization. It is important that community members know where and when immunization services are available.

10.4.1 Overcoming barriers to immunization

Immunization generally requires babies or young children to be injected and many parents have fears about this. The fears result from several factors, including a dislike of needles, and concerns about the transmission of HIV/AIDS or other health problems arising from the use of contaminated syringes and needles. Immunization injections can also cause reactions, such as a mild fever or pain in the injection site, and make the child cry. Mothers and families may thus be reluctant to follow the full course of immunization, or even to begin immunization, if other families have had bad experiences. *However, such reactions are not harmful to the child and the full course must be taken to ensure that the child is fully immunized.* Many rural families may feel they do not have the time to take children for immunization, particularly if immunization services are available only during periods of intensive work on the farms.

To overcome these barriers, immunization services should be available at times convenient for community members. Community leaders and health staff should also provide full information to families before immunization is started and ensure that everyone has an opportunity to ask questions and voice concerns. If immunization is to be effective, all children should complete the full course and obstacles to this must be overcome. Community meetings with health staff should help in overcoming such problems.

Figure 10.2 *Nurse immunizing a child*

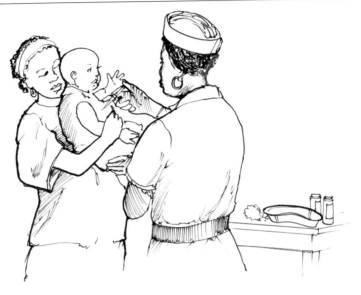

Checklist for immunization

- Are immunization services available at the local health centre?
- When are these services offered and who provides them?
- Are special arrangements required (e.g. do people have to make appointments; are there restrictions on how many immunizations can be done in one day)?
- If mobile teams offer immunization services, when will the services be available?
- Where will the immunization sessions be held?
- How many people can attend?
- Who is responsible for providing the community with feedback from immunization programmes?
- Has this information been provided?

While immunization should be carried out by trained health staff, the community itself has an important role to play in ensuring that this is done properly and that everyone has access to immunization services. It is important that the community receives information about how many children were immunized on each visit. A community health worker can be given responsibility for identifying families that have limited access to services or that do not use the services that are available. The health worker should then lobby for improved access and work with the families to persuade them to use the services available.

10.4.2 Making immunization safe

Immunizations are normally (and should be) carried out either at health centres or by mobile immunization teams. Immunizations requiring an injection should be carried out by qualified medical personnel, such as doctors or nurses; immunizations that are given orally (for instance poliomyelitis) can be given by other health staff under the supervision of a doctor or senior nurse. In all cases, the vaccines should be used before their expiration date. If disposable syringes and needles are used for vaccinations they should be safely discarded after use. A new type of safe, disposable syringe is now available, called the AD (auto-disable) syringe, which is much safer because it locks after a single use. Disposable syringes and needles are intended for a single use only and are highly dangerous if they are used more than once. If sterilizable syringes and needles are still used, they must be properly sterilized after each use to avoid the transmission of pathogens such as HIV, viral hepatitis B and hepatitis C. All used syringes and needles MUST be disposed of safely and not be left on the ground or in waste bins in the village, since they represent an extreme health risk, particularly for children who may find them and play with them. Preferably, needles, syringes and other medical waste should be taken away by trained staff and disposed of at properly designed facilities. If no such facilities are available, the waste should be incinerated or buried in the village but only if there is a secure site.

Several safety issues about which health staff need to reassure communities are listed in the text box below. Community members have a right to know the answers to these questions—they are important for establishing confidence in immunization services.

Safety issues for immunization programmes

- Do the people carrying out immunization have the necessary training?

- Are nonmedical staff supervised?

- Are the vaccines used by their expiry date? (Vaccines that have expired may lose effectiveness or become dangerous.)

- Are disposable needles used only once?

- Are sterilizable syringes and needles properly sterilized between injections?

- Are AD syringes available?

- How will used syringes, needles and other waste be disposed of?

10.5 Groups with special health care needs

Certain groups within a community will have special health care needs because they are more vulnerable to infectious or chronic noncommunicable diseases than the general population. These groups include the very young, the very old and pregnant women.

10.5.1 Pregnant women and infants

Local health care centres and village health care workers should provide advice and specialist care to infants and pregnant women. For infants, regular check-ups are necessary to ensure that they are not malnourished and are gaining sufficient weight. Children are particularly susceptible to infectious diseases that cause diarrhoea and extra care should be taken to ensure that water and food for children are hygienic. Parents, and particularly mothers, should actively encourage children at an early age to develop good hygiene practices, such as using latrines and washing hands.

Key checks for pregnant women

- Measure the growth and position of the baby.
- Test blood pressure.
- Test the urine for proteinuria.
- Perform blood tests for diseases such as HIV, syphilis and malaria, and to assess whether the mother is anaemic.
- Screen for women who will be at high risk for health complications and refer them to local hospitals for further checks and treatment. Those at high risk include women pregnant with twins, women who have previously had a caesarean section and women in their fifth (or greater) pregnancy.

Health care for pregnant women would usually be offered through a health centre or mobile health team. Antenatal and postnatal care are both vital for ensuring that mother and child remain healthy, and pregnant women should visit their doctor regularly for health checks. If basic antenatal and postnatal care are not available in a village, the community should lobby for such services to be provided. In areas where malaria is endemic, pregnant women should be given mosquito nets impregnated with insecticide as early in the pregnancy as possible.

10.5.2 The elderly

As people age they become more susceptible to ill-health, both from infectious diseases and from noncommunicable diseases, such as cancers or degenerative diseases. The risk of infectious disease is often increased by chronic disease, particularly when treatment involves treatment with certain drugs that can suppress the immune system and render it less effective. Some disabilities in old age may result from an earlier lifestyle and work, or from malnutrition and repeated infection in formative years. These disabilities can be prevented only by healthier lifestyles at a younger age.

Key illnesses that affect older people include heart complaints, strokes, eye problems (e.g. glaucoma), respiratory problems, deafness, arthritis, and problems with urinating and sleeping. If an elderly community member has eye or heart problems, he or she should visit a health centre and obtain treatment at an early stage of the disease. Many chronic health problems faced by the elderly either require long-term medication or have significant potential for recurrence. Planning for health care within the family and community may therefore require careful budgeting. Furthermore, many older people are sceptical of "western" or orthodox drug-based health care and it is important to make sure that they take their medication regularly.

If a community has a significant number of older people, it should lobby to ensure that the nearest health centre has someone with a particular interest in the care of the elderly and runs regular clinics dedicated to older people. Health education programmes that target the problems of the elderly and provide information on healthy ageing are often an effective way to improve the health and well-being of the elderly. Many older people also suffer from depression or anxiety as their physical abilities (such as eyesight and hearing) decline and they feel they are unable to contribute fully to the life of the home and community. To counter this, they should be encouraged to retain an active role in the community. While older people may not have the energy or strength to perform all the roles they used to, this should not mean that they are no longer asked to undertake important tasks. Indeed, their health and well-being may depend on being actively involved within the community. Developing a positive attitude towards ageing, among the young and old alike, will help people to remain active in later life and develop better support for the elderly.

10.6 Risky behaviour

Some people engage in behaviour that poses a high risk both to their health and to the health of their family. For example, if a person has sex with multiple partners and does not use condoms there is a high risk of contracting

HIV/AIDS and other sexually transmitted diseases. If the person is married or is in a relationship, he or she can then pass on the infection to their spouse or usual partner. This can have devastating consequences: infection with HIV can lead to the development of AIDS and to premature death, and other sexually transmitted diseases can cause infertility, problems during childbirth and stunting in babies.

Risky behaviour in a community

- Do people in the community engage in high-risk sexual behaviour?
- Do people in the community use drugs or drink too much alcohol?
- Is information about these problems available in health centres, schools or community centres?
- Is support available for people with drug or behavioural problems?
- Are community health workers aware of the health risks associated with these behaviours?

The abuse of substances such as alcohol, cigarettes and other legal and illegal substances, to the extent that an individual becomes dependent upon them, can also lead to severe physical health problems, such as liver dysfunction or cancer, and may make the person more vulnerable to heart disease and other health problems. Long-term use of such substances may lead to mental health problems or worsen existing problems. Dependence on a substance can also cause a person to neglect their normal social and family duties and take less care of their appearance. In some cases, people dependent on substances commit crimes in order to fund their habits.

10.6.1 Changing risky behaviour

People who engage in risky activities do so for many reasons, some of which may relate to other problems in their life or in their society. People who abuse substances or drink too much alcohol may do so not only to get a "buzz" or "high" but also because they have problems in their personal or family life or because they feel marginalized in their community. This behaviour can be a means of trying to cope with these problems. People who engage in high-risk behaviour do not always consider the impact of their behaviour on their own health and well-being, or on the well-being of their families and communities.

A first step in changing risky behaviour is to encourage people to talk about the impact that their behaviour has on themselves and on their community. This requires that they have access to information and support. Encouraging people to change risky behaviours takes effort and time, and may require working with individuals, households and the whole community. While it may be relatively easy to change a person's behaviour initially, sustaining such changes can be much more difficult. If a person reverts to the risky behaviour, it is important to continue to work with them and help them to stop the behaviour again.

One approach is to form a community support group with support from counsellors or other health personnel. Those engaging in risky behaviour can discuss the problems associated with their behaviour in terms of financial cost, losing respect, disharmony in the home and difficult interactions with neighbours. It is also important to identify the problems a person faces in trying to change their behaviour and to discuss factors that might encourage them to overcome these problems. This may require working with people to develop strategies for dealing with personal and family problems, and to develop other social and occupational activities in place of the risky behaviour.

Many people will need ongoing support and encouragement not to go back to risky behaviour. It is important not to penalize people who revert to risky behaviour; they should be helped to understand why they went back and encouraged to change. Such relapses can be used as a learning experience, helping the person to understand which situations trigger a return to risky behaviour. Eliminating this behaviour completely may not be possible and it may be more effective to keep it within limits that do not harm the person or their family. For example, drinking could be reduced to non-harmful levels. In some cases, the individual or community may need support from medical personnel or mental health specialists. Sometimes, when a person has become dependent on a substance, he or she will need medical assistance to stop using the substance. This is sometimes called "detoxification". Care should be taken to ensure that this process is properly supervised as it can pose a risk to health.

10.6.2 Health education

In addition to working with people who engage in risky behaviour, it is important to work with communities to develop strategies and knowledge for preventing it. As with many health issues, prevention is much better than trying to treat problems after they occur. Many of the techniques discussed in the previous chapter can also be used to raise awareness about risky behaviours. The whole community should be encouraged to participate in defining the impacts and problems associated with risky behaviours, and to discuss how they can be reduced or prevented.

It is especially important that children have access to information about the impact of risky behaviour on their health and on the well-being of their community. In this respect, health education in schools is very important and should be carried out in a way that allows children to openly discuss these difficult problems. In many areas, encouraging less risky sexual practices has proved to be an effective method for promoting better sexual health. In addition to school programmes, health centres and clinics should also be encouraged to provide information about the impact of risky behaviours. The information should be communicated in terms that are easily understood by the whole community, rather than in complicated medical terms, and community members should be provided with an opportunity to discuss issues with health staff. It is important, however, that such messages are not too harsh or strict. For instance, some consumption of alcohol may not be harmful and discouraging all use may be neither necessary nor helpful. It is more important to emphasize the need to keep consumption at levels that do not represent a risk to the person's health.

10.7 Mental health problems, learning difficulties and epilepsy

10.7.1 Mental health problems

Mental health problems are mental, emotional and behavioural difficulties that disrupt relationships and may impair the ability of a person to play a full and active role in the community. In some cases, mental health problems result from brain diseases, while in other cases they may be reactions to bad experiences. People with severe mental health problems often need to be given drugs to treat symptoms, but these can have side-effects that make people feel unwell or drowsy. As a result, some people stop taking their prescribed medication and feel they can cope without it, which can cause the illness to recur. People with mental health problems should therefore be encouraged to continue taking any medication that has been prescribed.

An important way to help people with mental health problems is to engage them in counselling or enrol them in mental health services. However, mental health specialists may not be easily accessible to community members, since there are usually relatively few of them, and they work at higher levels of service provision. To overcome this, community members should lobby for access or referral to mental health specialists or other health staff who can provide assistance, both in treating patients and in identifying support for the individuals and families. Assistance does not necessarily mean financial aid and often includes social support and health education. To help them feel valued within the community, people with mental health problems should be encouraged to take up employment and social opportunities.

10.7.2 Learning difficulties

People with learning difficulties have limited intellectual capabilities and may seem "slow", yet there are many ways in which they can play a meaningful role in their community. However, these people will often need support from their community and will benefit from input from health care and other staff, who can help them to develop their abilities and skills.

10.7.3 Epilepsy

People with epilepsy suffer from fits that can be alarming to themselves, their families and other community members. Epilepsy can be caused by head injuries during infancy, or result from maternal infections such as meningitis or syphilis. *Epilepsy is not an infectious disease and there is no risk of catching it from someone else.* Epilepsy can be treated and controlled with suitable medication, and when people with epilepsy are stabilized on medication they can play a full role in the community.

10.7.4 Social inclusion

People with mental health problems, learning difficulties or epilepsy are often stigmatized by the community because of ignorance about the nature of mental illnesses. This only compounds the problem by making those suffering from the illnesses and their families feel like "outsiders", and can lead to discrimination. Community members and health workers should work to overcome stigmatization and value the sufferers as full and useful members of the community. Often, this can be accomplished through education and by providing support services for these individuals. Encouraging them to undertake activities that are useful to the community, and that make them feel part of their community, can reduce the level of stigma and increase social inclusion. Schools should also include education about mental health to encourage greater understanding of the problems and of the ways in which sufferers can be supported to enjoy a full and productive life. Addressing problems of this nature with children often helps prevent stigmatization and other social problems, which are usually fuelled by ignorance.

Community mental health

- Are there people in the community suffering from mental health problems?
- Are there people in the community suffering from learning difficulties?
- Are there people in the community suffering from epilepsy?
- Are community health workers trained to provide support to these people?
- Does the community have access to mental health workers?
- What is the attitude of the community towards people with mental health problems, learning difficulties or epilepsy?
- Are educational materials about mental health problems, learning difficulties or epilepsy available to the community?

CHAPTER 11

Establishing committees for implementing Healthy Villages programmes

This chapter describes how to establish committees for Healthy Villages programmes and discusses the key roles of committees in implementing the programmes. It also provides an overview of the local and national government support that community leaders may expect when developing a Healthy Villages initiative. It is not meant as a definitive guide for government staff, as this is covered elsewhere (see Annex 2).

Healthy Villages initiatives usually extend beyond a single community or group of communities and are incorporated into provincial, district and national plans. Healthy Villages programmes are also often linked to similar programmes, such as Healthy Cities and Basic Development Needs. Each of the different programmes greatly benefits from close association with other programmes. For example, a Healthy Villages programme may be easier to run if the local urban area is engaged in a Healthy Cities programme. Thus, both national and local governments play key roles in supporting and developing Healthy Villages programmes.

Healthy Villages programmes in action

In the eastern Mediterranean region, Healthy Villages programmes have been integrated into national plans for improving health. In Egypt, for example, the Healthy Villages programme has been part of an integrated approach to rural development. By 1999, the programme had covered 4405 villages and satellite settlements in 1087 local administrative units. An estimated 36 million people (about 57% of the population) have benefited from the programme. A total of 25450 projects were implemented within five years in the economic, social and health sectors. A key lesson is that it is possible to integrate environmental and health concerns in a local development agenda and that this leads to greater stakeholder involvement.

11.1 The role of local community committees in Healthy Villages programmes

Each village and community participating in a Healthy Villages programme should establish a committee at the local level. Local committees are essential for broad approaches to health improvement that involve a wide range of activities and individuals, such as the Healthy Villages programme. A committee can coordinate and support the different activities and provide leadership for the community, and can serve as the community contact point with local and national government staff involved in the Healthy Villages programme. Local committees can also facilitate broad community participation in the programme, something that may be difficult to achieve by outsiders. Local committees are therefore crucial for promoting the Healthy Villages approach in a community.

11.1.1 Composition of a Healthy Villages committee

The composition of a local committee is critical for a successful outcome. Committee members should be influential people within the community who are respected and who are able to represent the interests of all the different community sections. If the committee reflects the narrow interests of only a small group of people, confidence may be lost in the entire programme, leading to failure. Ideally, the composition of the committee should reflect the gender balance of the community. While it may not be possible to have completely equal gender representation, because of cultural and social norms, women should be adequately represented to ensure that their concerns are taken into account and dealt with sensitively. It is also helpful if staff from the national or local government are members of the committee.

The importance of local committees in Healthy Villages programmes

Local village councils in the Islamic Republic of Iran have played key roles in the successful implementation of integrated rural development programmes. The strong role played by the local committees, supported with a legal mandate, has helped rural development programmes meet the demands of the local populations and deliver sustained improvements in public health.

The influential members of a community are not necessarily the people with administrative responsibilities within the community. They can also be people who are respected and act as opinion leaders, such as village chiefs, teachers, religious leaders and ordinary community members. It is best that committee members are elected by the community and have limited terms of office, to ensure that serving on the committee does not become a burden to key community members, or become a way for individuals to use the committee for personal gain. As the committee is expected to be the principal implementing body for the Healthy Villages programme, members must also have time to allocate to the committee and other Healthy Villages activities. They will also need to be accessible both to the community and to staff from local government and other bodies that provide support to the Healthy Villages programme.

11.1.2 Transparency and accountability

The committee should be accountable and transparent both to the community and to external organizations, such as local government, NGOs or external support agencies that may provide support. The committee should take minutes of all meetings, record the decisions made and make sure that other community members have access to this information. A regular feedback mechanism to the broader community should also be established, along with a forum for broader debate by the community about major activities and issues. If the committee manages funds, accounts should be kept and made available to other community members and external support agencies. To do this, the committee should elect executive officers, such as a chairperson, treasurer and secretary, and meet regularly.

11.2 The role of local government committees in Healthy Villages programmes

Local governments usually have their own Healthy Villages committees and coordinators who provide technical and administrative support to community committees overseeing Healthy Villages programmes. A key role of local government committees is to provide new ideas and to make communities aware of initiatives and successes in other communities participating in Healthy Villages programmes, and provide the impetus for communities to improve their own health and environment. For example, local governments may support improvements to communities under their jurisdiction by providing services and infrastructure. This may be paid for by local government revenue, by grants and loans from central government, or by raising funds from national and international support agencies. The delivery of many health services, such as immunization programmes or programmes that provide health centres and clinics, will be carried out by local government.

11.2.1 **Funding and accountability**

Often local governments have access to both conditional and unconditional grants for improving services to their populations. These grants can be used to support immunization programmes, for example, or provide funds for the operation and maintenance of water supplies and latrine construction. To retain access to these grants it is critical that local governments properly account for the funds. In most cases, central governments, external support agencies and NGOs are willing to provide continuing support to local governments if the funds are spent in accordance with agreements between the local governments and the finance providers and if all previously released funds can be properly accounted for. One of the greatest barriers to local governments accessing funds is an inability to properly account for money previously provided. This can result in local governments being blacklisted by agencies or central government departments, and lead to frustration within the local government and funding agencies over the inability to release funds.

In many cases, the lack of accountability does not reflect misappropriation of funds, but rather a lack of understanding of accounting procedures. It is essential, therefore, that local governments request proper training and support in accounting procedures, and ensure that their staff understand the accounting requirements and can prepare and submit accountability forms in the correct format.

11.2.2 **Technical advice and support**

In addition to providing infrastructure and services directly, local governments play an important role in other ways by providing support to communities in terms of technical advice, health education, water quality monitoring and management, lobbying for funds to support community-based initiatives, and facilitating access to spare parts and tools. Often, they can also support the development of health care provision within, or close to, communities. These different types of support can provide opportunities for educating community members on how to practise good hygiene, and how to improve the operation and maintenance of water supplies. Local governments can also provide services that the community is unable to deliver, such as periodic testing of wastewater quality, food inspection and food quality analysis.

Partnerships between communities and local governments

In Morocco, the rural water supply programme (PAGER) has developed close relationships between local rural governments (communes) and communities. The communes also provide a vital link to the national government. Rural water supplies have been developed through a partnership between the communes and local communities, with the communes providing technical support and advice. However, initiation of the process always comes from the local population.

Local government officials play a crucial role in providing technical advice to communities. Many communities or households may wish to facilitate better health by improving the environment, but do not know how to achieve this. Local government staff can provide technical advice on a wide range of activities, such as the design of sanitation, water supply, waste disposal and drainage projects, and work with communities to define and implement improvements that the community can afford and sustain. Local government staff willing and able to answer questions from community members can therefore assist in resolving many health problems.

Local government staff can also be the main implementers of health education by providing health education directly through community meetings, by providing posters, or by training and supporting local health educators. The use of community health educators, drawn from the community in which they live, can be a very successful approach if they are given adequate technical and financial support from local government. Local government staff also play a crucial role in helping communities to analyse their environment and the risks to their health, and in helping them prioritize interventions. They can also help communities use the checklists included in this document.

Finally, the local government can play a critical role in identifying the most needy communities and households, and in directing external agencies (whether large donors or NGOs) to those areas. This can ensure that all communities, rather than just a few lucky ones, receive equitable support and funds from Healthy Villages initiatives.

11.3 The role of national committees and coordinators in Healthy Villages programmes

A Healthy Villages programme usually has a national committee and a coordinator who are responsible for promoting and developing the programme at a national level. National committees help to articulate policies that support the development of Healthy Villages initiatives, and help to attract external support when required. They may also provide training for local government staff in techniques that are required to support Healthy Villages initiatives at local levels, to evaluate progress and to ensure that experiences are shared. To remain relevant, it is important that national committees remain in touch with developments in communities with Healthy Villages programmes and are aware of the reality of life in rural areas. They should also understand how community members want to develop their village. National staff should therefore make regular visits to villages participating in Healthy Villages programmes and listen to the views and concerns of local people.

The importance of national committees in promoting Healthy Villages programmes

To ensure that Healthy Villages programmes receive support, it is essential that there are national level professionals who are committed to the development of the Healthy Villages initiatives. In Egypt, the Islamic Republic of Iran, Jordan and the Syrian Arab Republic, the role of national committees in developing materials and attracting resources has been crucial. In all these countries, support from the highest levels of governments has been secured because of the profile and performance of these committees. A common factor across all these countries is that the national committees have maintained close contact with grassroots activities, thus ensuring that they remain responsive to the needs of the rural population and are well-respected.

National committees and coordinators are often responsible for the development of supporting materials that can be used by local Healthy Villages committees when undertaking a range of interventions. These materials can include overview guides for entire Healthy Villages programmes and concepts, or pamphlets and manuals on specific subjects, such as protecting and maintaining a water supply or improving sanitation and hygiene. Any materials developed should be properly tested before they are used and communities should be given opportunities to provide feedback on the usefulness of the documents and on changes that may be required.

National committees and coordinators should also make sure that lessons from different areas or countries with Healthy Villages programmes are shared with key stakeholders, including community leaders. Building on successes from other communities can be an important way for communities to improve their own programmes and avoid the mistakes of others. Consequently, community leaders should make sure that they know who the national committees and coordinators are, where they are located and what their roles are in developing a Healthy Villages programme. They should also request information about activities in other areas of the country, as well as those at the national level and in other countries.

Organizations supporting Healthy Villages initiatives

Many organizations, some of which are listed below, provide support for Healthy Villages projects at both local and national levels. Contact addresses are given only for WHO offices. For most other agencies it will be more effective to contact the corresponding country offices directly.

A1.1 Government ministries

- Agriculture.
- Cultural Affairs.
- Environment.
- Gender.
- Health.
- Labour.
- Water.
- Works.

A1.2 World Health Organization

The first step in discussing a Healthy Villages project is to contact a WHO office directly. WHO maintains offices in many countries, usually associated with the Ministry of Health. Addresses for WHO headquarters and regional offices are listed below. In most regional offices there are specific technical departments that deal with issues such as environmental health and they may be a valuable resource for information. Contact details for these departments should be obtained from the WHO country or regional offices.

- World Health Organization (WHO-HQ), 20 Avenue Appia, CH-1211 Geneva 27, Switzerland.
- World Health Organization, Regional Office for Africa (AFRO), PO Box No. 6, Brazzaville, Republic of Congo.

- World Health Organization, Regional Office for the Americas/Pan American Health Organization (AMRO/PAHO), 525 23rd Street, Washington, DC 20037, USA.
- World Health Organization, Regional Office for the Eastern Mediterranean (EMRO), WHO Post Office, Abdul Razzak A1 Sanhouri Street, Naser City, Cairo 11371, Egypt.
- World Health Organization, Regional Office for Europe (EURO), 8 Scherfigsvej, DK-2100 Copenhagen Ø, Denmark.
- World Health Organization, Regional Office for South-East Asia (SEARO), World Health House, Indraprastha Estate, Mahatma Gandhi Road, New Dehli 110002, India.
- World Health Organization, Regional Office for the Western Pacific Region (WPRO), PO Box 2932, 1099 Manila, Philippines.

A1.3 **Other United Nations organizations**

The following organizations often have a national office in countries:

- United Nations Children's Fund (UNICEF).
- United Nations Development Programme (UNDP).
- United Nations Environment Programme (UNEP).

In addition, there are bilateral donor agencies (agencies that are the official body for a single country), multilateral donor agencies (agencies that represent a group of countries, such as the European Union) and international lending institutions, such as the World Bank, and these may also support a Healthy Villages project.

A1.4 **Nongovernmental organizations (NGOs)**

Many NGOs may be able to provide technical or financial support to a Healthy Villages programme. Information should be sought about which NGOs (national or international) are active in a country, and whether they would be willing to provide support. Some examples include:

- African Medical Research Foundation (AMREF).
- Action contra la Faim (ACF).
- CARE.
- CONCERN.
- Federation of Red Cross and Red Crescent Societies.
- GOAL.
- Helen Keller Foundation.
- International Rescue Committee (IRC).

- Médicins Sans Frontières (MSF).
- OXFAM.
- Save the Children Fund (SCF).
- WaterAid.

ANNEX 2

Books and manuals providing further advice

Almedom AM, Blumenthal U, Manderson L. *Hygiene evaluation procedures: approaches and methods for assessing water- and sanitation-related hygiene practices*. London, International Nutrition Foundation for Developing Countries, 1997.

Byrne M, Bennett FJ. *Community nursing in developing countries: a manual for the community nurse*, 2nd ed. Oxford, Oxford University Press, 1986.

Cairncross S, Feachem RG. *Environmental health engineering in the tropics: an introductory text*, 2nd ed. Chichester, England, Wiley, 1993.

Boot MT. *Just stir gently: the way to mix hygiene education with water supply and sanitation*. The Hague, Netherlands, IRC International Water and Sanitation Centre, 1991 (IRC Technical Paper Series, No. 29).

Boot MT, Cairncross S, eds. *Actions speak. The study of the hygiene behaviour in water and sanitation projects*. The Hague, Netherlands, IRC International Water and Sanitation Centre, 1993.

Ferron S, Morgan J, O'Reilly M. *Hygiene promotion: a practical manual for relief and development*. London, Intermediate Technology Publications, 2000.

Franceys R, Pickford J, Reed R. *A guide to the development of on-site sanitation*. Geneva, World Health Organization, 1992.

Guidelines for drinking-water quality. Vol. 1: Recommendations, 2nd ed. Geneva, World Health Organization, 1993.

Guidelines for drinking-water quality. Vol. 3: Surveillance and control of community supplies, 2nd ed. Geneva, World Health Organization, 1997.

Hofkes EH, ed. *Small community water supplies*. Chichester, England, Wiley, 1983.

Howard G. *Water quality surveillance—a practical guide*. Loughborough, England, Water Engineering and Development Centre, Loughborough University, 2002.

Hubley J. *Communicating health: an action guide to health education and health promotion*. London, Macmillan, 1993.

Jordan TD. *A handbook of gravity-flow water systems for small communities*. London, Intermediate Technology Publications, 1984.

Kolsky P. *Storm drainage: an engineering guide to the low-cost evaluation of system performance*. London, Intermediate Technology Publications, 1998.

Mara D, Cairncross S. *Guidelines for the safe use of wastewater and excreta in agriculture and aquaculture: measures for public health protection*. Geneva, World Health Organization, 1989.

Mariotti SP, Prüss A. *Preventing trachoma—a guide for environmental sanitation and improved hygiene: the SAFE strategy*. Geneva, World Health Organization, 2000 (document WHO/PBD/GET/00.7/Rev.1).

Morgan P. *Rural water supplies and sanitation: a text from Zimbabwe's Blair Research Laboratory*. London, Macmillan, 1990.

Pacey A, Cullis A. *Rainwater harvesting: the collection of rainfall and runoff in rural areas*. London, Intermediate Technology Publications, 1986.

PHAST step-by-step guide: a participitory approach for the control of diarrhoeal disease. Geneva, World Health Organization, 1998 (Participatory Hygiene and Sanitation Transformation Series; document WHO/EOS/98.3).

Quick RE et al. Diarrhoea prevention in Bolivia through point-of-use water treatment and safe storage: a promising new strategy. *Epidemiology and Infection*, 1999, **122**:83–90.

Rozendaal JA et al. *Vector control: methods for use by individuals and communities*. Geneva, World Health Organization, 1997.

Safe water systems for the developing world: A handbook for implementing household-based water treatment and safe storage projects. Atlanta, GA, Centers for Disease Control and Prevention, 2000 (available at www.cdc.gov/safewater/manuals.htm).

Sobsey MD. *Managing water in the home: accelerated health gains from improved water supply*. Geneva, World Health Organization, 2002 (document WHO/SDE/WSH/02.07).

Stern P, ed. *Field engineering: an introduction to development work and construction in rural areas*. London, Intermediate Technology Publications, 1985.

Surface water drainage for low-income communities. Geneva, World Health Organization, 1991.

Water for health: taking charge. Geneva, World Health Organization, 2001 (document WHO/WSH/WWD/01.1).

Watt SB, Wood WE. *Hand-dug wells and their construction*. London, Intermediate Technology Publications, 1979.

Werner D. *Where there is no doctor: a village health care handbook*. London, Macmillan, 1983.

Werner D, Bower B. *Helping health workers learn: a book of methods, aids and ideas for instructors at the village level*. Palo Alto, CA, The Hesperian Foundation, 1982.

Williams T, Moon A, Williams M. *Food, environment and health: a guide for primary school teachers*. Geneva, World Health Organization, 1990.

Date Due

NOV 1 1 2003			